HEAD INJURY

Information and Answers
to Commonly Asked Questions

A Family's Guide to Coping

HEAD INJURY

Information and Answers to Commonly Asked Questions

A *Family's* Guide to Coping

CHRISTOPHER D. STURM, M.D.
Division of Neurosurgery, Department of Surgery, Saint Louis University
Health Sciences Center, St. Louis, Missouri

THOMAS R. FORGET, Jr., M.D.
Division of Neurosurgery, Department of Surgery, Saint Louis University
Health Sciences Center, St. Louis, Missouri

JANET L. STURM, R.N.
Neurosurgical Intensive Care Unit, Saint Louis
University Hospital, St. Louis, Missouri

ILLUSTRATORS
Sharon Harris, M.A.M.S. • Joel Harris, M.A.M.S.

Quality Medical Publishing, Inc.
ST. LOUIS, MISSOURI
1998

PUBLISHER   Karen Berger
EDITOR   Beth Campbell
PROJECT MANAGER   Katherine Spakowski
PRODUCTION   Susan Trail
BOOK DESIGN   Diane Beasley
COVER DESIGN   Diane Beasley

Quality Medical Publishing, Inc.
11970 Borman Drive, Suite 222
St. Louis, Missouri 63146
Telephone: 1-800-348-7808
Web site: http://qmp@qmp.com

LIBRARY OF CONGRESS CATALOGING-IN-PUBLICATION DATA

Sturm, Christopher D.
     Head injury : information and answers to commonly asked questions :
a family's guide to coping / Christopher D. Sturm, Thomas R. Forget, Jr.,
Janet L. Sturm : illustrations Sharon Harris, Joel Harris
          p.   cm.
     Includes bibliographical references and index.
     ISBN 1-57626-096-8
     1. Brain damage—Popular works.   2. Brain damage—Miscellanea.
I. Forget, Thomas R.   II. Sturm, Janet L.   III. Title.
RC387.5.S785   1998
616.8—dc21   98-28737
                                                                 CIP

QMP/BC/BC
5   4   3   2   1

Contributors

REV. SCOTT K. DAVIS, M.Div.
Director, Clinical Pastoral Education, Department of Pastoral Care,
Saint Louis University Hospital, St. Louis, Missouri

AMANDA L. HOFFMEISTER, M.S.W., L.C.S.W.
Senior Social Worker, Department of Social Work, Saint Louis
University Hospital, St. Louis, Missouri

SR. ANN JOHNSTON, O.P.
Staff Chaplain, Department of Pastoral Care, Saint Louis
University Hospital, St. Louis, Missouri

REV. GREGORY KIRSCH, M.Div., M.A.
Staff Chaplain, Department of Pastoral Care, Saint Louis
University Hospital, St. Louis, Missouri

CHRISTOPHER KUSELIAUSKAS, R.N.
Nurse Specialist, Department of Neurology, Saint Louis
University Hospital, St. Louis, Missouri

ELISABETH PRICE, Ph.D., M.A.
Staff Chaplain, Department of Pastoral Care, Saint Louis
University Hospital, St. Louis, Missouri

To

All those families
whose courage and questions
helped make this book
possible

Preface

The purpose of this book is to provide some general information and answers to commonly asked questions regarding the various aspects of head injury, particularly severe head injury. While there is no question that such an injury is a tragedy, understanding some of its facets may help those who find themselves suddenly and unexpectedly dealing with it. It became clear through our interactions with head injury patients and their families that such a reference source would be valuable. Unfortunately, the time a physician can spend with family members explaining the various issues may be limited.

This book is not meant to replace the physician-patient-family relationship but rather to supplement that interaction. By providing a source of information designed for families dealing with the tragedy of head injury, family members will hopefully be better equipped to discuss matters with their physician and manage the crisis in a somewhat enlightened manner. Head injury typically strikes suddenly without warning and with significant impact, both to the patient and the family. Family members are often left in a state of shock, filled with a multitude of questions regarding the injury, its implications, and prognosis. This book is designed to address those questions and explain, in layperson's terms, what all the beeping and buzzing from the various machines really means.

Each chapter in this book begins with a few pages of facts and information about the different aspects of head injury. We have tried to avoid being too technical, since this book is designed for the general public and not physicians. However, we thought that a knowledge of certain medical terms was necessary to adequately explain the issues and to facilitate communication between family members and health care providers. To this end, terms in **bold type** within the text are briefly defined in a glossary of the most common medical terms, procedures, and concepts.

To avoid gender conflicts, the injured individual is referred to as "the patient" in both the text section as well as the section of commonly asked questions that is part of each chapter. Some chapters have more questions than others, with the chapters on head injury management having the most. For those looking for answers to specific questions, a listing of all the questions is included at the end of the book. These questions have been gathered from years of experience working with these patients and their families. Although it is not likely that every question is addressed, the collection is representative of the questions most often asked by families. Again, the explanations are general in nature and designed to be easily understood, but clarification should be sought from a physician or nurse involved in the care of a particular patient.

Excerpts from interviews with family members who found themselves confronting this sudden tragedy of head injury have also been scattered throughout the text. Their individual stories are introduced in Chapter 1. These interviews illustrate that no one is alone in the fear, confusion, concern, and desperation that surround these devastating injuries.

In addition to the information addressing the various medical and surgical issues of head injury, information from pastoral care personnel and social workers has been included. These professionals are intimately involved with family members as they cope with the consequences of such injuries. Regardless of a family's religious preference or social situation, it is hoped that these chapters will add to the book's usefulness as an informational reference. Various rehabilitation issues are also discussed.

While we realize that nothing can ever totally prepare a person for the devastation caused by a brain injury to a loved one, we hope that this book will aid family members to gain an understanding of the issues at hand and provide reasons why the health care staff is "doing what they are doing." Our hope is that, with this information and knowledge, some of the fear and confusion will dissipate and communication between family members and the medical team will be more rewarding.

Christopher D. Sturm, M.D.
Thomas R. Forget, Jr., M.D.
Janet L. Sturm, R.N.

Acknowledgments

This book would not be a reality had it not been for the help from some outstanding people at Saint Louis University Health Sciences Center. As with any topic, multiple viewpoints enrich the discussion. In an attempt to provide these varied points of view, we sought out contributions from individuals involved in different aspects of care of the head injury patient. The time and expertise of the nurses, social worker, pastoral care personnel, and rehabilitation specialist give this book its unique flavor. Certainly, the book would be incomplete without their contributions.

The many commonly asked questions included in these pages are the result of the concerted efforts of Lisa Kuciejczyk and Diane Reynolds, two nurses on the front line in our neurosurgical intensive care unit. Their input regarding these questions helped to form the core of this work.

Amanda Hoffmeister provided the information on issues confronting the social worker. Countless numbers of patients, and their families, have relied on her experience in coordinating and facilitating posthospital discharge arrangements. Her contribution to this text should prove to be a valuable resource.

The pastoral care aspects were developed through the combined efforts of Elisabeth Price, Sr. Ann Johnston, Rev. Gregory Kirsch, and Rev. Scott Davis, who deal with the emotional and spiritual concerns of family members confronting the tragedy of head injury on a day-to-day basis. Their insight into the suffering and concerns of these family members is commendable.

The rehabilitation aspects of care were provided by Christopher Kuseliauskas, whose experiences with neurological rehabilitation proved to be an invaluable resource. We have seen first hand the functional recovery made possible by Chris and his coworkers in head injury patients.

Connie Pickering, research coordinator for the National Acute Brain Injury Study (Hypothermia), and Beth Campbell, our editor at Quality Medical Publishing, Inc., arranged and conducted the family interviews. Encouraging these family members to recount the emotional landslide that they experienced was greatly facilitated by Connie and Beth's gentle manner and understanding.

We would like to especially thank the family members who participated in the interviews. Although reliving their experiences was traumatic, each embraced the idea of giving insight to other family members in crisis. That willingness to discuss a most terrible event in their lives demonstrates the courage that these people possess.

The editorial support provided by Edward Matthews was invaluable in putting this work together and his colorful comments still bring smiles to our faces. Hopefully, there are still smiles on the faces of Joel and Sharon Harris of Articulate Graphics, our illustrators, who weathered the many discussions we had regarding the images with good humor and professionalism.

This book would not have been possible without the continued support from our mentor, Kenneth R. Smith, Jr., M.D. Thank you.

Finally, our own family members, especially our parents and spouses, provided the encouragement, patience, and understanding that gave us the strength to continue with this project. This book would never have been completed were it not for their constant love and support.

Contents

Part I

THE ACUTE PHASE: THE HOSPITAL EXPERIENCE

Part II

THE NEXT STEP: REHABILITATION

PART

I

THE ACUTE PHASE

THE HOSPITAL EXPERIENCE

1

The Accident:
Three Women Share
Their Stories

Each year in the United States, approximately half a million people suffer a head injury severe enough to require hospitalization. Of these people, about 50,000 die before they get to the hospital. Fortunately, most of the survivors have mild injuries, which have a better outlook for a good recovery. However, approximately 20% have either moderate or severe head injuries. These more serious injuries are associated with both increased disability and likelihood of death. To compound the situation, 70% of the patients with a severe head injury have other traumatic injuries, which adds to the severity of the patient's overall condition.

As illustrated by the above statistics, head injury is relatively common. Patients with varying degrees of injury are regularly seen in most neurosurgical intensive care units, especially those in medical centers that handle a large number of traumatic injuries. Overall, trauma is the leading cause of death in people under 45 years of age. The likelihood of a death from an accident increases when head injury occurs as part of the traumatic injury. One study of trauma patients suggests that a patient is three times as likely to die if head injury occurs in combination with the other traumatic injuries sustained at the time of the accident.[1] In 1990 there were 148,000 recorded injury-related deaths in the United States. In approximately half of those fatalities, it was thought that the primary reason for death was due to serious brain injury.[2]

Head injury is most commonly seen in young men, with the peak incidence occurring between the ages of 15 and 24 years.[2] The leading cause of such injury in the United States is motor vehicle accidents. Falls, gunshot wounds, and assault are also major causes. Another contributing factor to traumatic head injury is alcohol intoxication, with an incidence as high as 72% in those involved in accidents leading to head injury.[2]

INTERVIEWS
Donna and Sharon

Donna is the sister of Sharon, a middle-aged woman who sustained a severe head injury as the result of a motor vehicle accident. Although Sharon did not require surgery, her medical course was very difficult and complicated. However, she has made a remarkable recovery considering the severity of her injury.

> **Donna:** We had planned a "girls' weekend" at the lake. We were meeting at my house on Friday afternoon, but Sharon was late. It was about 1:00 and I kept saying, "She should be here by now, something's wrong. She had a flat tire, or broke down, or something." Finally, another friend, Pam, and I went looking for her. She was nowhere to be found.
>
> I was frantic and used the cell phone to call both my house and her house. I knew something had happened. We stopped at my house and she wasn't there, so we went to her house, which is just a few blocks down the road. Her mother-in-law was there. She said, "Sharon was in an accident." She said Sharon had been taken by helicopter to a nearby university hospital. I broke down. We all raced to

the hospital, which is nearly 45 minutes by car. It was the longest ride of my life.

In our search we had driven right past the accident site, but they had already cleared the wreckage. . . . The road was slick and she had hit a tree by the bike trail where we used to walk together every-day. A cop was sitting in the parking lot of the bike trail and wit-nessed the accident. He thinks she was probably in a little bit of a hurry, saw him, hit the brakes, and slid. She hit the tree with the dri-ver's door directly up against the tree. So her head was right there.

Sarah and Jim

Sarah, the wife of a farmer, related the story of how her husband sustained an open head injury after being hit on the head with a tree branch. His injury was also considered to be severe. Jim re-quired emergency surgery for a depressed skull fracture and a blood clot within his brain. Although his recovery has been slightly ham-pered by a seizure, he has done quite well since the accident.

Sarah: My husband was on a tractor clearing a tree for a fence line. He was pushing on the dead tree and a limb above fell off and hit him on the head. It wasn't even that big of a limb. . . . He was knocked unconscious but I don't think he was in a deep coma. Our son, Josh, who was nine years old at the time, and Jim's brother, Bob, were with him at the time of the accident, helping him clear the tree. Thank goodness it was a weekend and they were there; no telling what would have happened if he had been alone.

Immediately after the accident, Bob quickly drove from the pas-ture to the house and said, "Call 911!" I was in the yard playing ball with our daughter and I panicked. Jim was still on the tractor, kind of slumped back. Josh stayed there with him. Jim looked to be asleep; there was no blood or mark of any kind.

I rode along in the ambulance to the local hospital. When they said they were taking him by helicopter to a bigger hospital, I freaked.

Ellen and Steve

Ellen is the mother of 18-year-old Steve who sustained a severe head injury after a rollover motor vehicle accident. Ironically, the patient's father had died 15 years earlier from a head injury he had sustained in a car accident. Steve had a severe head injury yet experienced a relatively rapid recovery. Such a quick recovery should be viewed as the exception, rather than the rule, in discussing severe head injuries.

> *Ellen: Steve didn't have much experience driving on a major interstate. Although he had been driving for almost two years, it was mainly around town. He had just been to a job interview and had gotten the job. He was coming home on the highway, near a construction site. All we know for sure is that there was a car parked on the shoulder of the road, and it looked like he swerved to avoid it, lost control, flipped several times, and hit a concrete median head-on. The median had just been poured and they said it had some "give." That essentially saved his life. It's a miracle that he got out alive.*
>
> *Ironically, my first husband, Steve's father, died about 15 years ago from a head injury he received in an automobile accident. The difference was that he was hit in the back of the head. He was in a coma for 10 days and then died.*
>
> *I was at home when I found out about Steve's accident. My other son, who was at school waiting to be picked up by Steve, called and said, "Mom, he's not here yet." I thought, "Oh, that stupid car." They had just put in a new engine so I said, "I bet he's stuck on the road somewhere. Wait 15 minutes and I'll go look for him." My neighbor called all upset and said, "I just passed a terrible accident, I think it's Steve." She recognized his car. I called 911 and said I wanted a ride to the hospital. Their response was, "Ma'am, we don't do that. You'll have to find your own transportation." I just couldn't think of what else to do. Then the hospital called me. By that time I was hysterical. The woman from the hospital said it was a head injury and he was in critical condition. It was kind of dejá vu. My two*

youngest children were at home with me, and I thought, "My God!, I can't let them see me so upset." I didn't know what to do. I waited until my husband, Larry, came home; it seemed like forever, although I think it was about 20 minutes at the most. Larry had passed the accident on his way home. He noticed it but thought nothing of it. You never think it will happen to someone you know and love. By the time we got to the hospital, an hour later through rush hour traffic, we were both shaking. We didn't know what we were walking into.

The accident changed Steve's life. It changed mine, too. My biggest problem is that I'm a nervous wreck. If my husband or any of the children are a few minutes late, you know . . . I have to get over it. I try to think it's never going to happen again, but I know that it can.

REFERENCES

1. Gennarelli TA, Champion HR, Sacco WJ, et al. Mortality of patients with head injury and extracranial injury treated in trauma centers. J Trauma 29:1193-1202, 1989.
2. Kraus JF. Epidemiology of head injury. In Cooper PR, ed. Head Injury, 3rd ed. Baltimore: Williams & Wilkins, 1993, pp 1-25.

2

Understanding the Brain and How It Works

Basic Anatomy

THE BRAIN AND BRAIN STEM

The brain, also called the **cerebrum,** is extremely complex and, despite the many discoveries that have advanced our knowledge of the brain, many aspects of its function still remain a mystery.

The brain is encased in a thick protective membrane called the **dura.** Inside this sac of dura lies the brain, which floats in a clear fluid called **cerebrospinal fluid** or **CSF.** The skull encases this sac and provides further protection against brain injury. The brain itself is divided into halves or **hemispheres** (Figure 2-1). Each hemisphere is then further divided into portions called lobes. In general, each lobe has a different set of functions, all of which are interconnected to make us who we are. The lobes are paired, such that there is a left and a right one. The **frontal lobes** are located in the front of the brain, just behind the forehead. The **temporal lobes** are located on the sides of the brain, just behind the temples. The **parietal lobes** are immediately behind the frontal lobes, toward the back of the head, and the **occipital lobes** are located the farthest

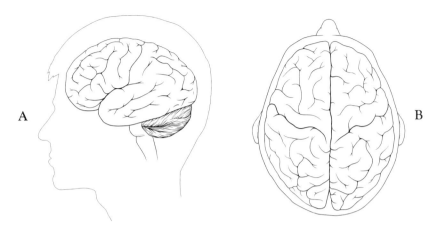

Figure 2-1   A, A side view demonstrates the general orientation and position of the brain and brain stem within the head. The brain actually "floats" in the CSF contained within the dura. **B,** A view from above looks down on the brain (i.e., cerebrum). The brain is divided into two halves called hemispheres. Each hemisphere is further divided into portions called lobes.

from the frontal lobes in the back of the head (Figure 2-2). The **cerebellum** lies underneath the occipital lobes in its own bony compartment called the **posterior fossa** (Figure 2-3). This is a special compartment within the skull located at the junction between the skull and the neck. The roof of the posterior fossa is made up of thick fibrous tissue called the **tentorium,** which separates the cerebellum from the occipital lobes.

The brain, with all its interconnected lobes, communicates with the body via two "relay stations," the **thalamus** and **brain stem** (Figure 2-4). Both organize and convey messages between the brain and the other parts of the body. The thalamus, which sits on top of the brain stem, is intimately connected with all the portions of the brain. This acts as a "filter" or "traffic cop" for messages, directing the correct pathways for the signals to travel. The brain stem consists of three different subdivisions: the **midbrain** (the uppermost portion of the brain stem), the **pons** (just below the midbrain), and the **medulla** (lowest portion of the brain stem).

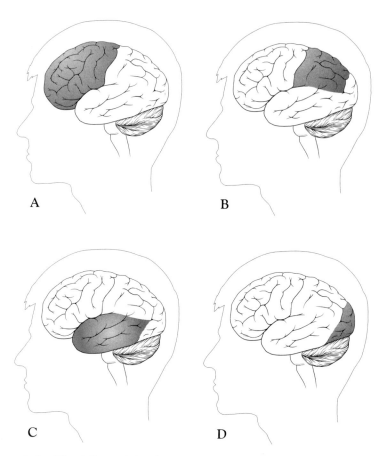

Figure 2-2 The different lobes have been shaded. **A,** The frontal lobe. **B,** The parietal lobe. **C,** The temporal lobe. **D,** The occipital lobe.

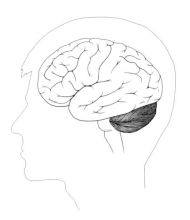

Figure 2-3 The cerebellum sits in the posterior fossa and is separated from the cerebrum by a thick fibrous layer called the tentorium.

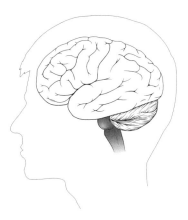

Figure 2-4 The brain stem is divided into the midbrain, pons, and the medulla. It forms the connection between the brain and the spinal cord as well as coordinating many important functions.

THE VENTRICLES AND VESSELS

The brain is made up of protein, fat, and millions of cells. These cells require nutrients, oxygen, and a method of waste-product disposal to survive. Any interruption in either the nutrient supply or disposal mechanism can lead to dysfunction of the brain. The brain has its own internal plumbing system through which CSF and waste products flow. This system, called the **ventricular system,** is located within the center of the brain (Figure 2-5). CSF, which is made in the ventricles, flows through this system and ultimately exits the brain. The ventricular system is composed of interconnected compartments. The uppermost and largest portion of the ventricular system is called the **lateral ventricle,** of which there are two, a left and right. These funnel into a smaller single chamber below, called the **third ventricle.** The third ventricle then empties into another small single ventricle in the cerebellar compartment called the **fourth ventricle.** The drainage pipe connecting the third ventricle with the fourth ventricle is called the **cerebral aqueduct,** a very small tube that can easily become blocked, causing a backup of the plumbing system and a buildup of pressure within the brain.

While the ventricles bathe the brain in CSF, the various cerebral blood vessels provide the much-needed oxygen and nutrients carried in blood to the cells of the brain. Think of the blood vessels as a set of pipes that branch into different segments enabling blood and oxygen to flow into the various parts of the brain. The **internal carotid artery** is the main "pipe" carrying blood with oxygen and

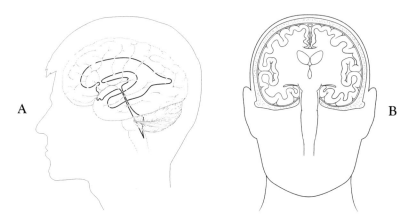

Figure 2-5 **A,** The ventricular system is located deep within the brain. This system, which contains the CSF, consists of the lateral ventricles, the third ventricle, cerebral aqueduct, and fourth ventricle. The CSF flows through these ventricles and then leaves the brain to enter the space surrounding the spinal cord. **B,** A view from the front depicts the location of the ventricles within the center of the brain. The surrounding dura and skull can also be seen.

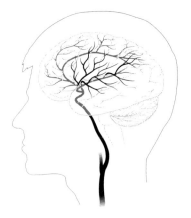

Figure 2-6 The branches of the internal carotid artery. The internal carotid artery travels up through the neck, then branches into the anterior and middle cerebral arteries within the brain. These vessels further divide into smaller vessels that supply blood and oxygen to the brain. The vertebral-basilar artery system is not shown.

nutrients from the heart to the brain. This is the largest artery that supplies blood to the brain and is the one whose pulse you can feel in the neck under the jaw. This artery travels into the brain and then splits into two main branches, the **anterior cerebral artery** and the **middle cerebral artery.** The anterior cerebral artery travels toward the front of the brain (the frontal lobes), then loops upward and backward along the top of the brain. The middle cerebral artery travels out along the side of the brain (Figure 2-6). There is another separate, paired set of arteries that supply the brain. These are called the **vertebral arteries,** which enter the brain from the back of the neck and then combine into one artery called the **basilar artery,** which is an important artery that supplies blood to the brain stem.

⚜ COMMONLY ASKED QUESTIONS ⚜

Where is CSF made?

CSF is made within the ventricles. Small structures located within these fluid-filled spaces, called the **choroid plexus,** continuously make small amounts of this clear fluid. After it is made, the CSF flows within the interconnected ventricles and eventually out of the brain into the space around the spinal cord. The CSF is then absorbed into the bloodstream after flowing around the spinal cord and surface of the brain. The amount absorbed is roughly equal to the amount produced. This acts to maintain a general balance between the amount made and the amount removed from the CSF space. This is why the ventricles do not normally enlarge despite the fact that CSF is continuously being produced within these structures.

Where does the CSF go after it leaves the brain?

Once the CSF is made, it first flows through the various ventricles. For example, CSF made in the lateral ventricles will flow into the third ventricle. From there the CSF flows down through the cerebral aqueduct into the fourth ventricle, located near the cerebellum. The CSF then flows out of the fourth ventricle and into the space around the spinal cord. This space, which runs all the way down the back, is thus normally contiguous with the ventricular system. The CSF makes its way down and around the spinal cord and then percolates up over the surface of the brain. It is here that the CSF is absorbed into the bloodstream. Thus CSF leaves the inside of the brain, flows around the spinal cord, and then flows over the outside of the brain where it is subsequently absorbed into the blood.

Why does the patient produce so much CSF?

Normally the ventricles produce small amounts of CSF continuously. Within a 24-hour period the ventricles renew the total CSF volume, comprised of both the brain and spinal cord CSF spaces, approximately three times. This is one reason patients with CSF leaks can continue to leak CSF throughout the day. In the normal situation, CSF is also continually absorbed into the bloodstream as new CSF is made by the ventricles. The CSF is absorbed after it leaves the ventricles, flows around the spinal cord, and finally up and over the surface of the brain. The CSF system is now in balance since the amount of CSF produced is approximately equal to the amount absorbed into the blood. In the absence of injury or abnormality, this system acts to bathe the brain and spinal cord in the continually fresh supply of CSF.

Head injury can disrupt this normal balance. The presence of blood clots in or around the ventricles, as well as any nearby compression, can result in blockage of the normal CSF pathway. When such an obstruction is present, the CSF begins to build up in the ventricles. This leads to enlargement of the ventricles called **hydrocephalus.** Hydrocephalus can also occur if the normal CSF absorption mechanism on the surface of the brain is disrupted. Blood located on the brain's surface can result in such a blockage. As the CSF continues to be made in the absence of normal absorption, the ventricles also begin to enlarge. In both of these abnormalities, which result in hydrocephalus, the disruption of the normal CSF pathway and absorption mechanism leads to the problem, not the amount of the CSF being produced. This amount remains relatively the same.

Where is the brain stem located?

The brain stem is located on the bottom of the brain in the center. It forms the connection between the brain and the spinal cord below. This is analogous to what a mushroom looks like, the cap is the brain and the stem is the brain stem. In addition to forming the connection between the brain and spinal cord the brain stem also serves several important functions. Two of these are the life control center and the ascending reticular formation, which plays a role in maintaining consciousness. Because of its location, the brain stem can become compressed by the surrounding swollen brain. **Herniation** can be the result if this compression is significant.

What is the brain made of?

The brain is an incredible feat of nature. This "natural computer" remains far more complex than anything present technology has been able to develop. Even more amazing is the fact that this incredible complexity is carried out by millions of cells called **neurons** with a multiplicity of connections. The brain in essence consists of millions of cells made up of various proteins and fat. During development each cell makes many connections with other cells in the brain and spinal cord. These cells and their connections form the basis for all the various functions that the brain and spinal cord control. Our personality, memories, ideas, hopes and desires, and movements and sensations are the product of the combined actions of these cells and their connections.

Where are the different lobes located?

The brain is divided into two halves, the left and right. These halves are called the cerebral hemispheres. Each hemisphere is divided into four different portions called lobes. These are the frontal, temporal, parietal, and occipital lobes. The frontal lobes, as the name implies, are in the front of the brain. The temporal lobes are immediately behind and slightly below the frontal lobes (these lie underneath the area on the head known as the "temple"). The parietal lobes are located immediately behind and above the frontal lobes. The occipital lobes are located in the back of the head, below the parietal lobes. The cerebellum lies underneath the occipital lobes in a special compartment in the skull.

What protects the brain from injury?

The brain is protected by various layers of tissue. The skin (i.e., the scalp) is the first level of defense and helps to protect the skull and brain, particularly from infection. The second layer of defense is the skull, which completely encases the entire brain. The hard bone of the skull provides formidable protection against impact. Infants and young children, however, have less protection against impacts because the skull at this stage of life is not fully solidified. The third layer of protection is provided by the dura. The dura is a very tough fibrous sac that surrounds the brain. Contained within this sac is the CSF in which the brain floats. The dura acts to both protect the brain from impact as well as protect the brain against infection. The CSF contained within the dura also acts as a fluid cushion protecting the brain from impact. These multiple layers of protection act to prevent injury to the brain from incidental impact-type injuries as we grow up. Typically significant forces, such as those involved in motor vehicle accidents, are required to breach these lines of defense and produce brain injury.

What is the function of the cerebral arteries?

The cerebral arteries supply blood and oxygen to the various areas within the brain. The oxygen carried in the blood is necessary to keep the neurons (brain cells) alive and functioning properly. An interruption of the normal blood flow to an area within the brain can lead to cell death if it is not reversed within 4 to 7 minutes. There are two pairs of arteries that supply the brain with blood.

The internal carotid arteries supply the majority of the brain with blood while the vertebral arteries supply the brain stem and a small portion of the brain.

If a vessel is torn or occluded, will it cause brain damage?

Cerebral blood vessels serve the important function of supplying blood and oxygen to the tissues of the brain. There are two pairs of vessels that supply the brain with the necessary blood and nutrients. The two internal carotid arteries represent the main blood supply to the brain. These arteries divide into smaller branches once they enter the brain, which deliver blood and oxygen to a large portion of the brain tissue. The other pair of vessels are the vertebral arteries. These arteries, which run through the cervical neck bones up into the back portion of the brain, supply blood to the brain stem and a small area in the back of the brain. Tearing or occluding (i.e., stopping blood from flowing through the artery) one or more of these vessels can result in a stroke. This occurs when an area of brain does not receive enough blood and, subsequently, enough oxygen and the cells begin to die.

However, this is not always the case in these types of injuries. In a certain percentage of patients, the internal carotid artery and vertebral artery systems are interconnected, which provides a backup blood supply system for the brain and brain stem. For example, although the normal blood flow through one of the internal carotid arteries may be interrupted, a stroke can be prevented if the other internal carotid artery picks up the slack. Due to the fact that the blood supply systems are connected, the opposite side internal carotid artery can supply blood to the brain that was originally supplied by the injured internal carotid artery. The vertebral artery system also has this capability. The question as to whether a stroke will occur in any given patient with interrupted blood flow through an artery depends on how well the remaining vessels can take up the slack. Older patients who typically have some degree of arteriosclerosis have a much more difficult time with this than younger patients with healthier blood vessels.

Brain Function

Ultimately, it is the *function* of the brain that is important, not only to the patient, but also to the family members who worry about the degree of severity and the permanence of any functional loss their loved one may have suffered as a result of the injury. It is the preservation of function that is the aim of all the intensive management utilized in the care of head injury patients. While there are some generally agreed upon locations for various functions, it should be understood that many functions rely on the interplay of various areas within the brain. Furthermore, locations for various functions may be in different areas in different patients. For example, while many individuals have speech functions located in the left parietal and frontal lobes, some patients have speech functions located in the right side of the brain. In addition, even though a particular function should be lost with an injury to a particular area, the brain can sometimes get around this loss of function and compensate with other healthy areas of the brain. The result is that the anticipated loss of function due to injury of a particular portion of the brain does not manifest itself. Keeping these ideas in mind, the following is a very simplistic description of where certain functions are located.

DOMINANT VERSUS NONDOMINANT BRAIN

The brain is conceptually divided into a **dominant** and **nondominant** side. This division, based primarily on the location of speech function, is also referred to as the "left" or "right" brain. Most people have the function of speech located on the left side of the brain, particularly right-handed individuals. Even those who are left-handed usually have speech functions located on the left side of the brain. The other side of the brain, usually the right side, deals with functions other than language. Typically these relate more to the artistic aspects of life, such as music appreciation or painting. Injuries to the right side of the brain usually, but not always, do not result in language and speech deficits.

FRONTAL LOBES

The frontal lobes are considered to be the parts of the brain responsible for our more human qualities (Figure 2-7). The abilities for complex thinking, planning for the future, motivation, emotions, and the awareness of what is right and wrong within the confines of a given society are located in the frontal lobes. The summation of these functions results in the individual's personality. The frontal lobes also serve the important function of motor control for the body, including control of the muscles used in producing speech. It is here that the decision and the commands for the body to move originate. This includes control of some eye movements. The manner in which the brain and the body are wired results in the right side of the brain controlling the left side of the body and face, and conversely for the left side. This is also true for sensory and visual functions.

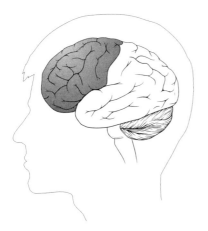

Figure 2-7   The frontal lobe.

TEMPORAL LOBES

The temporal lobes (Figure 2-8) are mainly concerned with memory function. They help store new memories and may be involved in the retrieval of old ones. The dominant temporal lobe (again, usually the left) is also involved in the ability to understand as well as formulate speech. This function is controlled in conjunction with the dominant parietal lobe. Although not a function of the temporal lobe, the visual impulses from the eyes to the "vision" parts of the brain (the occipital lobes) run through a portion of the temporal lobes as well. This is important because injuries to the temporal lobes, while they are not involved in the control of vision, can damage these connections and result in partial visual loss (see Chapter 6).

PARIETAL LOBES

The parietal lobes (Figure 2-9) help to interpret the world around us through sensations, such as touch, vibration, and pain, which are relayed to the brain from the body. The parietal lobe on the dominant side (usually the left side of the brain) plays a significant role in language interpretation. It also enables us to form complete, coherent sentences, as well as read and write. It is from this lobe that the messages on how and what to say are sent to the frontal lobe. The frontal lobe then tells the muscles involved in the actual production of speech to carry out the program (to say what it is we want to say). Similar to the temporal lobe, a portion of the connection from the eyes to the occipital lobe (involved in the function of vision) runs through the parietal lobe.

OCCIPITAL LOBES

The occipital lobes deal primarily with vision (Figure 2-10). While the eyes actually gather the images, much the way a lens does on a camera, the occipital lobe interprets, or "develops," the film into images that are then recognizable. As with motor and sensory func-

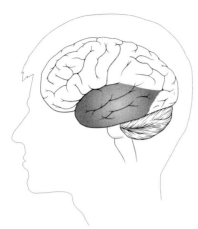

Figure 2-8   The temporal lobe.

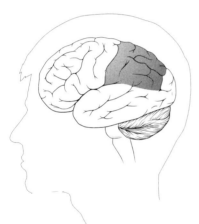

Figure 2-9   The parietal lobe.

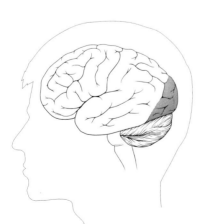

Figure 2-10   The occipital lobe.

tion (served by the frontal and parietal lobes, respectively), the **visual system** is also **crossed,** such that the images collected by the right eye are sent to the left occipital lobe and the right occipital lobe receives images collected by the left eye. The two sides of this visual system act in combination to provide a three-dimensional view of the world.

CEREBELLUM

The cerebellum is concerned with coordination. As we walk, talk, move a part of our body, or just stand still, the cerebellum is constantly correcting and fine-tuning the muscles of our bodies to provide balance and smooth movements.

BRAIN STEM AND THALAMUS

As already described, the brain stem and thalamus form the connection between the brain and the body. Several other important functions are also located in the brain stem (Figure 2-11). The system responsible for maintaining consciousness, as well as waking us from sleep, called the **ascending reticular activating system** or **ARAS,** runs through the upper portions of the brain stem. The midbrain (the uppermost portion of the brain stem), in conjunction with the pons, helps to control eye movements so that they move together, termed **conjugate gaze.** The midbrain also helps to control the size of the pupils. Other portions of the pons control the blink reflex, termed the **corneal reflex,** which helps to protect the eyes from dirt and keeps them lubricated. Perhaps the most important portion of the brain stem is the medulla. It is here that the "life control center" is located. Areas that control automatic functions that keep us alive, such as breathing, blood pressure control, and heart beating, are located within this structure. The protective **gag reflex,** which helps to prevent food from going down the wind pipe **(trachea)** and into our lungs when we swallow, is also controlled by the medulla.

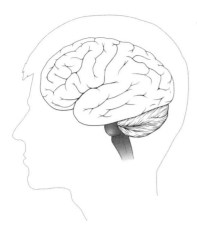

Figure 2-11   The brain stem. The thalamus (not depicted) lies immediately above the brain stem.

———❧ COMMONLY ASKED QUESTIONS ❧———

Upon awakening, will the patient be able to walk, talk, and see?

The functions that are available to the patient upon recovery depend on which areas of the brain were injured and to what extent those injuries caused irreversible injury. The brain, unlike the skin or other organs, does not grow back. The key to this question is whether the injury produced permanent damage to the brain and the extent of that damage. There are areas in the brain, such as the frontal lobes, that can be extensively damaged with little or no effect, while in other locations, such as the brain stem, very small areas of damage can result in a serious disabling loss of function. Another factor is the patient's ability to compensate for the loss of function (i.e., other parts of the noninjured brain may make up for damaged areas that typically were responsible for a given function). Younger patients' brains can compensate for areas of lost function better than older patients.

Keeping in mind that many areas of the brain are often involved in different functions, there is some general information regarding the ability to walk, talk, and see. The frontal lobes are involved with the ability to move, including the ability to walk.

Walking is actually very complex. The patient must first be awake enough to get into a position to walk; therefore, the portions of the brain that are responsible for consciousness and leg movement cannot be irreversibly damaged. The cerebellum, which is responsible for coordination, must work properly to allow for a smooth coordinated gait, as well as for the ability to stand up without falling (i.e., balance).

Language ability, as with walking, is also a fairly complicated function that relies on different portions of the brain to work properly. In most people, the language part of the brain is on the left side, so patients with damage to the left side of the brain have an increased likelihood of having some degree of speech problem. The left parietal, frontal, and temporal lobes are particularly important in dealing with the ability to speak and to understand speech. Irreversible damage to these areas may result in the complete or partial loss of the inability to speak or understand speech.

The capability to see relies on the eyes being intact, the occipital lobes remaining relatively undamaged, and the connections between the eyes and the occipital lobes remaining intact. It is unusual to completely lose the ability to see, but it can happen if there is extensive irreversible damage to both eyes or both occipital lobes. More commonly, a patient may lose the ability to see a portion of the visual field but this is typically something that the patient can learn to overcome.

Will the patient remember me?

Many of the patients with significant head injury have a certain degree of **amnesia** (a period of time in which the patient does not remember what occurred), particularly for the actual accident and the events that took place while unconscious in the **intensive care unit** or **ICU**. This is actually a blessing, as the events of the injury are often traumatic, and having tubes and wires attached while in the ICU can be an unpleasant experience.

Memory is stored throughout the brain and, although much of this process is not fully understood, it is thought that the temporal lobes are involved in the process of making new memories. Irreversible damage to both temporal lobes could result in the inability to make any new memories. With regard to long-term memories, or memories that have already been stored, the patient may initially have difficulty remembering anything. As the brain begins to heal and the patient awakens, old memories typically return, including the ability to recognize people that the patient knew for a long time prior to the accident. However, this return of memory may take awhile and the memories that the patient had prior to the accident may not all return. Think of it as the brain "resetting" after the injury, much the way a computer must upload all its memory after first turning it on. This resetting of the brain and all its functions can take a variable period of time and, although it usually occurs, it may be incomplete, depending on the amount of damage that occurred in the brain.

According to where the injuries are located, what deficits should I expect?

Each patient is unique in that injuries in one area may produce a particular deficit, while in another the same type of injury results in a different deficit. The degree to which a particular deficit exists also varies among patients. For instance, one patient may not be able to move the left arm at all, while another with a similar lesion may only be slightly weak in the affected arm. There are, however, general locations for particular functions, and damage to these areas can result in some loss of function.

In most patients the left side of the brain is concerned with language function. This includes the ability to read, write, speak, and understand speech. Most of these functions are located in the left parietal lobe. Damage to this area can result in an inability to understand speech and perform other language functions called **aphasia.** Another type of aphasia can occur with damage to the left frontal lobe in which the patient may be able to understand speech but is unable to respond. The patient is actually unable to make the words with the mouth and vocal cords. The result is garbled speech, as if the patient had a mouthful of marbles. In these cases, patients can usually read and write, so they can communicate with a notepad. Speech therapy is usually quite successful with this type of difficulty, and patients can often overcome this deficit to some degree.

The frontal lobes are also involved with the motor control of the body. Damage to the areas within the frontal lobe that control movements in the body can result in weakness or a complete inability to move the affected limbs if the damage is severe enough. The brain is wired so that injury to one side of the brain results in a deficit in the opposite side. Damage to the right frontal lobe can result in weakness in the left side of the body. The deficit in movement can affect either the face, arm, or leg. The weakness can also be in all three areas if the damaged area is large enough. Together, the frontal lobes are also involved in emotion, personality, motivation, and the development of new ideas. Severe damage to both frontal lobes can result in blunting of the personality and a loss of motivation. Patients with such injuries appear very flat and emotionless and are typically quiet.

Damage to the temporal lobes can affect the ability to store new memories, while older memories formed prior to the injury are usually retained. It is uncommon to completely lose the ability to make any new memories, but patients with injury to the temporal lobes, particularly both temporal lobes, have a harder time remembering new facts. In general, patients with a head injury have difficulty with concentration and the performance of complicated tasks. The degree to which this deficiency remains after recovery is dependent on the severity of the head injury.

Although damage to the cerebellum can result in loss of coordination and unsteadiness, this problem usually improves with physical therapy and time. The loss of coordination can affect any movement made by the body, including the eyes. Patients with damage to the cerebellum may have **nystagmus,** a condition where the eyes appear to jump around or rhythmically beat toward one side. Although very distracting to the patient, this usually also resolves with time.

Since the patient is not moving his or her arms and legs now,
will he or she ever be able to move them?

Patients may not move for many different reasons. Depending on
the etiology of the immobility, the length of time that the patient
remains motionless can vary. Patients may not move because they
are deeply unconscious. While these patients typically do not move
spontaneously, significant stimuli (such as deep pain) may elicit a
response. Responses in these types of patients tend to be the more
stereotypical **posturing** movements. The fact that the patient is
able to move in some way indicates that the "movement connections" are intact to some degree, despite the damage that caused the
unconsciousness. In the absence of any new injury, patients who
demonstrate movement on both sides of the body generally retain
that ability as they recover.

Patients who are receiving chemical **paralytics,** such as Norcuron, will not move as long as the medication is being administered.
This lack of movement is not necessarily due to any injury but
rather secondary to the medication, which paralyzes the muscles.
These patients cannot move, and thus there will be no response despite multiple types of stimuli. This effect dissipates as the medication is discontinued. Patients who do not have damage to the
movement control centers in the brain or brain stem should be able
to move once the medication's effect has disappeared.

Patients with injury to the **motor cortex** (the area in the frontal
cortex that controls movement) may have either weakness or complete **paralysis** on the opposite side of the body. This may affect a
single limb, such as the arm or leg, or the entire side of the body
may be involved. Patients who are unable to move an entire side of
the body are said to have **hemiplegia.** The weakness or paralysis in
these situations is typically only on one side. This may be permanent if the damage to the area is severe enough. This same type of
deficit can also occur with injury to certain areas in the brain stem.
Extensive damage to both sides of the brain stem or a cervical
spinal cord injury can produce the inability to move either side of
the body. This is called **paraplegia** and is often permanent. While

extensive damage to both frontal lobes could theoretically result in paraplegia, such an event is a rare occurrence in head injuries.

What part of the brain is considered the "real person," or the personality portion?

An individual's personality is most likely a summation of multiple events and experiences that have occurred throughout the person's life. The particular way an individual acts and reacts in different situations is likely the result of the interplay between many different areas within the brain. It would be extremely difficult to ascribe a patient's personality or "real person" characteristics to one particular area within the brain. The frontal lobes, however, are considered to be an area in the brain in which many personality characteristics are located and integrated. Some patients with extensive damage to the frontal lobes have been noted to develop personality changes. These often manifest as a depressed motivational drive that can be so extreme that the motivation to eat and move are absent. Injuries to the frontal lobes can also produce other types of personality changes, such as decreased inhibition, loss of the sense of what is right and wrong, and depression. Due to the complexity of any individual's personality, it is very difficult, if not impossible, to predict the effects that damage to the brain will have in terms of the patient's personality. For example, one patient may have no personality changes from a particular injury, while another may show definite changes from the same type of injury.

Another factor to consider is the major role language function plays in our day-to-day interactions. Speech and language are the methods we use to express ourselves. Injuries that result in the inability to understand or produce speech can significantly affect a patient's interactions. Patients who have a significant difficulty with speech function may become agitated as they become increasingly frustrated in their attempts to communicate. Other patients may be very depressed when they are not able to speak or understand speech. Hence, many factors play a role in how a patient responds and acts after head injury.

What is the difference between short-term and long-term memory?

Memory can be generally divided into two types: short-term and long-term. Memory is the storage of events and facts for later retrieval. Events and information to be stored get plugged into the memory storage mechanism. These stored items are first considered to be short-term memories. We tend to remember these things because they have just happened. The information in this short-term memory storage is constantly being turned over as we are bombarded with new information. At some point, if the brain decides that the information is valuable enough to retain for longer periods of time, it moves into the long-term memory storage area. Information placed here is retained for a very long period of time. An example of a long-term memory is recalling a family member who died many years ago. A short-term memory may be remembering what was just ordered at a restaurant. Most likely, this will be forgotten in a week or so, rather than moved into long-term memory.

Which side of the brain is the dominant side?

The dominant hemisphere refers to the side where speech and language functions are located. In the majority of patients the dominant hemisphere is the left side. Anatomical studies have indicated that most patients who are right-handed have language function located in the left side of the brain (i.e., the left hemisphere). The majority of the left-handed patients also have language function located on the left side. Some patients who are left-handed, however, may have language and speech function located in the right hemisphere. This is why the health care staff often asks whether the patient is right- or left-handed. The location of the language function has implications in terms of whether particular areas of damage are likely to produce language function impairments. This is also a consideration when surgery is being contemplated because neurosurgeons tend to be less aggressive in treating damaged areas located in the left hemisphere (especially in right-handed patients) so as to preserve as much language function as possible.

What happens if the dominant side of the brain is injured?
What about the nondominant side?

The dominant side of the brain refers to the location where speech and language function is located. This is the left hemisphere in the majority of patients. Damage to the dominant hemisphere can produce speech deficits called aphasias. The different types of aphasias are each produced by damage in different areas within the dominant hemisphere. These speech deficits can be divided into two general groups: the inability to understand speech and the inability to produce the sounds that make up the speech. Damage to the dominant parietal lobe (i.e., usually the left parietal lobe) can lead to the inability to understand speech. Patients may be unable to communicate because they do not understand anything that is said to them. They often also have significant difficulty reading and writing. While these patients can produce the sounds that make up speech, they cannot get the words straight or in the correct order. In other words, the words they say sound normal but the content of what they say often does not make sense.

Damage to the dominant frontal lobe (again, usually the left one) can lead to the inability to actually make the correct sounds we interpret as speech. While these patients are able to understand what is said to them, they cannot respond appropriately because they cannot get their vocal apparatus to function properly. These patients appear tongue-tied, or speak as if they have marbles in their mouth. Unlike patients with damage to the dominant parietal lobe, however, these patients can read and write appropriately.

Damage to the nondominant side of the brain, by definition, does not result in speech abnormalities. As is true with damage to either side of the brain, injury to the nondominant side of the brain can result in movement, sensory, and visual deficits. These patients may also have difficulty telling the difference between the left and right side of the body, as well as performing simple tasks, such as getting dressed.

What can we expect to see with a parietal injury?

The effects of injury to the parietal lobes depend on which parietal lobe is injured. Injury to the nondominant parietal lobe, usually the right, can result in sensory loss on the opposite side of the body. Another possible effect from such an injury can be partial loss of vision in a half or quarter of the visual field. There is also a set of clinical signs referred to as the "nondominant parietal lobe syndrome." In this syndrome the patient may ignore the left side of the body, thus having difficulty performing simple tasks. Damage to the dominant parietal lobe, usually the left, can result in sensory loss on the right side of the body and visual loss as well. One major disability that can result from dominant parietal lobe lesions is a problem with speech. The patient may have difficulty using and understanding spoken words.

Another problem common to all cortical brain lesions is the development of seizures after a traumatic injury. Therefore, damage of either parietal lobe may cause the patient to have seizures.

How will the patient's vision be affected by an occipital injury?

Injuries to the occipital lobe can cause deficits in the opposite visual field. This system is arranged so that an injury to the left occipital lobe will affect the right visual field. Think of the visual field as a large clock face. Each eye has its own field of vision that is essentially circular. When we look out both eyes at the same time, we see our complete visual field. An injury to the left occipital lobe can result in loss of the right half of the visual field. To use the clock analogy, the area from 12 o'clock to 6 o'clock will not be seen. If both occipital lobes are injured, the patient may be unable to see at all despite having eyes that are perfectly normal. This is referred to as cortical blindness and is similar to a camera with no film in it.

If the injury to the occipital lobe also involves the **corpus callosum,** the patient may lose the ability to read in addition to the visual field loss. The corpus callosum helps connect the two sides of the brain, including the two occipital lobes. Injury to the corpus callosum in this area can result in a disconnection between the visual areas (i.e., the occipital lobes) and the vocabulary centers located in the parietal lobes, leaving the patient unable to read.

Will the visual deficit be in one or both eyes?

Most injuries that result in some type of visual loss affect both eyes. The visual loss, however, is typically incomplete in that only a portion of the visual field is affected. For example, damage to one of the temporal, parietal, or occipital lobes can result in a partial visual field loss. This occurs secondary to damage to the connections between the eyes and the occipital lobes (the part of the brain that processes the visual information obtained by the eyes) as the impulses travel through these different lobes on their way to the occipital lobes. Such injuries do not result in complete blindness in either eye. The exception is when there is injury to a single optic nerve. The optic nerve leaves the back of the eye, carrying the visual information toward the occipital lobes. If this nerve is cut or irreversibly damaged, the affected eye will be completely blind. The same is true for irreversible damage to the eyeball itself. The unaffected eye will continue to function normally enabling the patient to see out of that eye.

Is the vision problem temporary or permanent?

It is often difficult to predict the severity and the permanency of a visual loss. Typically patients with head injuries are too confused to fully cooperate with the complex tests needed to accurately assess vision. When the patient is unable to speak or communicate effectively, recognizing a visual problem is difficult.

An injury that causes complete disruption of the eyeball itself or transection of the optic nerve will cause permanent visual loss in the affected eye. Irreversible injury to the eyeball, such as complete disruption of the globe, may require surgical enucleation (removal) of the eye. In these cases the patient will obviously not be able to see out of that eye again.

What will we see with a cerebellar injury?

The cerebellum is our balance and coordination center. Injuries to the cerebellum may result in problems with balance or with performing precise tasks. Many patients will sway to one side when they walk or have trouble feeding themselves because they are unable to perform the precise movements necessary. These difficulties usually improve with therapy and time.

One extremely serious consequence of cerebellar injury is related to the cerebellum's close proximity to the brain stem. The cerebellum is located in the posterior cranial fossa. This is a small, relatively compact area located in the back of the head. The brain stem lies immediately in front of the cerebellum. When the cerebellum is injured, it may swell or hemorrhage and become displaced in a forward direction. The posterior cranial fossa is so small that even a small amount of swelling or blood can cause the cerebellum to push into the brain stem, which is a very delicate and extremely important structure. Compression of the brain stem, due to swelling in the cerebellum, can be fatal in a matter of seconds.

Why is the brain stem so important? What does it control?

The brain stem is an extraordinarily important structure, controlling a large number of complex vital mechanisms. The centers for respiratory drive, heart rate control, consciousness, swallowing, and eye movement coordination are all located in the brain stem. Almost every part of the brain stem contains a vital center. Its most important function is the maintenance of an adequate heart beat, breathing rate, and blood pressure, which is controlled by the medulla. The brain stem, in conjunction with the thalamus, plays a role in the maintenance of consciousness as well. In addition to these two very important functions, the brain stem also controls various reflexes. These include the **pupillary reflex,** in which the pupils get smaller in response to bright light and larger when there is little light, thus optimizing the amount of light that reaches the eye when we are trying to see something; the corneal reflex, which causes the eye to blink when the surface of the eye is irritated, thus protecting the eye; a reflex that helps to move the eyes in tandem as they are moved from side to side and up and down, thus providing a three-dimensional view of the world while preventing double vision; and the gag reflex, which causes an individual to gag if the back of the throat is irritated, thus protecting the airway from inadvertent aspiration. The brain stem also contains all the pathways that carry information to and from the brain. These include commands from the brain to the body telling particular limbs to move and impulses from the body to the brain carrying sensations, such as pain, temperature, vibration, and touch. Because so many important functions are controlled by the brain stem, and damage to this structure is often irreversible, such injuries have very serious consequences. For example, brain stem compression from herniation can rapidly lead to death or irreversible coma.

When you test the brain stem functions, what are you looking for?

Brain stem function plays many important roles. The most important is the life control center located in the medulla. This center, which helps to control breathing, heart rate, and blood pressure, is crucial to maintain life. Additional areas within the brain stem control other important functions as well, including various reflexes that act to protect the patient. Due to the importance of this structure, brain stem function is continually checked. By testing various aspects of the brain stem's function, the health care team can assess the relative health of the individual brain stem centers. By determining the presence or absence of particular functions, the health care team can make an estimation of the extent of the brain stem's injury. This same information can also be used to subsequently follow the progression and clinical course of that damage.

In addition to monitoring the patient's overall condition, determination of brain stem function is also instrumental in assessing unconscious patients. Patients can be unconscious either because of brain injury or brain stem damage. It is important to differentiate between the two because brain stem injuries tend to be more critical. Assessment of brain stem function is also used to determine if the life control center is in jeopardy. The initial injury can begin to expand, either within the brain stem itself in patients who suffer brain stem damage at the time of the accident, or secondary to compression from the swelling brain. Evidence of extensor posturing (**extending**) and lack of a gag reflex indicates that the area of damage within the brain stem is very close to the life control center. Further extension of the injury into this center can quickly lead to the patient's death. While relatively little can be done for the injury located within the brain stem, various treatments can help to decrease brain swelling and subsequent compression of the brain stem. By closely following the patient's brain stem function, the health care team can determine if those various treatments are being effective.

Can a patient lose all brain stem functions and still be awake, alert, and alive?

Patients who lose all brain stem functions do not survive. Damage to the life control center can cause the patient to permanently stop breathing, stop the heart from beating, and, subsequently, result in the lack of any blood pressure. This situation is not compatible with life. This illustrates that, while the brain stem does not play a role in higher thinking, it does play a crucial role in life support. Injuries to the brain stem that spare the life control center usually do not result in death but they can produce significant alterations in consciousness, in the ability to move and feel, and in the ability to move the eyes. A fairly rare injury can occur in which the higher functions located within the brain are fully operational (i.e., the ability to think or understand speech) and the patient is awake but unable to move any part of the body, including the eyes and face. This unfortunate condition is called the "locked in syndrome," in which the patient appears to be deeply unconscious and immobile but is actually completely awake.

CHAPTER
3

Types of Head Injury

There are many different types of head injury, some more severe than others. The severity of the patient's injury is dependent on the type, extent, and location of the damage sustained at the time of the accident. For example, a person hit on the forehead with a baseball may have a lump but be neurologically unaffected. The same person may sustain a fatal injury if hit in the temporal area with the same baseball traveling at an identical speed. It is not always the size of the damage that determines the severity of the injury. The location of the injury within the brain plays a significant role. A small area of injury in the brain stem can be devastating to the patient, while a larger area of damage in the frontal lobe may leave the patient with minimal deficits. In addition, certain people may be more resistant to head injury than others. Not uncommonly, in a serious automobile accident with multiple passengers, there will be fatalities as well as passengers who sustain little more than a scratch. This variability in injury severity and the patient's response to the injury plays a role in the overall outcomes for these patients.

As previously stated, the skull contains the brain, blood vessels, and the **ventricles.** Any or all of these structures may be damaged by a blow to the head. The skull is an extremely important defense against brain injury. However, it can also be responsible for many of the injury patterns seen in the brain. There are two general types of head injury: closed head injury and open head injury. **Closed head injury** refers to a force delivered to the skull that causes some degree of brain injury without damaging the skull. Although the skull is not fractured or damaged, the brain injury inside can be very serious. **Open head injury** occurs when the force imparted on the skull causes a fracture of the skull bones. The broken pieces of skull may be driven into the brain. In these cases the brain may actually be visible in the wound. This type of injury often requires surgery because an opening in the skull can lead to a very serious infection. The bacteria normally living on the skin can get into the opening and begin to grow in the wounded brain.

INJURIES TO THE BRAIN PARENCHYMA (TISSUE)
Concussion

This is the mildest form of head injury. A concussion refers to a head injury in which a person loses consciousness for a brief period of time (about 3 to 5 minutes). In effect the brain is momentarily stunned. After this brief period of unconsciousness, the patient awakens but has no loss of function. Typically the patient has a headache and some degree of amnesia (the patient does not remember) for the events surrounding the actual accident. These patients usually have a normal **computed tomography** or **CT** scan of their brain.

Brain Contusion

A **contusion** is a bruise to the substance or parenchyma of the brain. This occurs from direct impact to the head. Remember, the brain essentially floats inside the skull in a pool of **cerebrospinal fluid** or **CSF.** When a person is traveling at a high rate of speed (i.e., in a car), the person's brain and body are also traveling at that speed. If the car suddenly hits something, there is an immediate de-

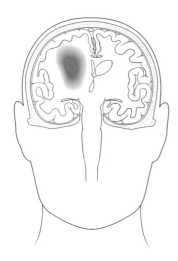

Figure 3-1 View from the front depicts a cerebral contusion. A cerebral contusion is essentially a "bruise" within the brain tissue that can begin to swell and compress the adjacent areas. Note the compressed ventricle on the same side of the contusion.

celeration of both the car and the patient, and the brain, due to the fact that it is essentially floating within the skull, crashes into the inner walls of the skull. Essentially the brain is stopped by the skull. This skull/brain impact causes damage to the more fragile brain tissue (Figure 3-1).

The site and severity of the brain injury depend on the velocity and the location of the impact. Common sites for contusions are the **frontal** and **temporal lobes.** The undersurface of the frontal lobes and the tips of the temporal lobes are especially vulnerable to such contusions because during rapid deceleration they can be raked across the irregular inner surface of the skull. Contusions can also occur on the complete opposite side of the impact. This is called a "contra-coup" injury. An example of such an injury is the development of a contusion in the back of the brain despite getting hit in the front of the head. Large contusions may require surgical removal.

Laceration

The brain laceration occurs when the brain is cut or torn apart, usually by some object driven into the head. Such injuries are typi-

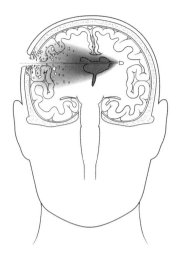

Figure 3-2 A gunshot wound. The large amount of damage produced by these injuries occurs as the bullet tears through the brain, leaving a "wake" of destruction behind its path. Bone fragments are often driven into the brain when the bullet pierces the skull.

cally very serious. Penetrating injuries, such as a gunshot wound to the head, can cause extensive damage and lacerations to the brain tissue. Such penetrating injuries destroy both the brain and skull as the object (i.e., a bullet) causes direct tearing of the brain as it passes through the tissue (Figure 3-2). A second cause of laceration is in an open skull fracture in which the in-driven bone can tear the brain and surrounding blood vessels. These injuries generally require surgery to clean the wound and remove any foreign debris in an attempt to prevent possible infection. Surgery may not be an option if the extent of the injury is such that the patient is so badly injured neurologically that an operation would be ineffective in reversing the tremendous damage done to the brain. This is often the case with high-velocity gunshot wounds to the head.

Shearing

In order to understand this concept it is important to appreciate that the brain is not a rigid structure. It is rather soft and is essentially a gelatinous ball of millions of interconnected nerve cells. When a person is struck on the head, the head and brain turn away from the impact. This turning or twisting causes rotational forces to develop within the brain. These rotational forces are similar to the pressure applied when wringing out a wet washcloth. The twisting causes incredible pressure on the nerve fibers in the brain and often leads to overwhelming loss of brain cells and their connections. This leads to very extensive and diffuse brain injury. These shearing-type injuries can be one of the more devastating injuries. Patients with this type of injury may be **comatose** indefinitely.

Cerebral Edema (Brain Swelling)

For all its differences, the brain responds to injury in much the same way as any other part of our body. Everyone has experienced the pain of a stubbed toe or a thumb struck with a misdirected hammer. The thumb becomes red and swollen, sometimes growing to two or three times its original size. Swelling occurs after injury because the body sends special chemicals and cells to the injured area to help repair the damage. This cellular response occurs on a microscopic level, but the results can be easily seen by the naked eye. This swelling is not unique to thumbs and toes. The cells of the brain act in a similar fashion, sending many types of "rescue cells" and substances to help repair damage. These cells are a kind of double-edged sword; while they act to help repair damaged areas, they can also cause significant **cerebral edema** or brain swelling.

This can be very harmful due to the resulting increased pressure inside the brain. Remember, again, that the brain is rather soft and floats in a sea of fluid inside the rigid skull. Unlike a thumb or toe, which can swell indefinitely, the brain has nowhere to go as it begins to swell within the skull and, in effect, the brain begins to push in on itself. The pressure within the skull begins to increase as the swollen brain begins to push on the surrounding unyielding bone of the skull. The increased pressure, called **intracranial pressure** or **ICP,** can cause further damage by directly compressing vital areas of the brain. The increased pressure also acts to inhibit the normal blood flow to the brain, leading to further brain cell death and strokes. Controlling brain swelling (or cerebral edema) is a major concern for the neurosurgeon treating head injury. Many times special monitoring devices must be inserted inside the skull to directly measure the intracranial pressure. This can be done in the intensive care unit (ICU) and is a great help in treating these patients.

Herniation

Herniation, while not another type of brain injury in the strictest sense, is rather a secondary effect of various primary brain injuries. The word herniate means protrusion of a bodily structure through the wall that normally contains it. Brain herniation refers to an event in which a portion of the brain is pushed or swells out of its normal location.

As described earlier, the brain is divided into three main parts: the **cerebral cortex,** the **cerebellum,** and the **brain stem.** The brain stem, located in the lower middle aspect of the brain, is where the life control center is located. This center controls the heart rate, breathing, and blood pressure and thus is crucial for life. Any compression of this area can lead to damage and ultimately death to the patient. Keep in mind that the brain is very soft, having the consistency of firm Jell-O. This and the fact that the brain does not completely fill the skull allows the brain to be pushed to one side by any damaged area that is swelling. As contusions or expanding blood clots begin to enlarge, these areas begin to the push the brain around within the skull. Similarly, in situations where the entire brain is swollen or the ICP is very high, the outer portions of the brain (which are pushed up against the skull) begin to compress the inner parts of the brain. As the brain begins to shift within the skull cavity, areas not initially injured may become compressed. This compression can lead to damage of these normal portions of the brain.

Once the compression of the brain (either by an expanding damaged area or by elevated ICPs) reaches a significant level, the brain stem is pushed. As the abnormally swollen brain surrounds the brain stem, it begins to strangle it. The blood supply to the brain stem is compromised (i.e., decreased secondary to the compression on the brain stem blood vessels), which can lead to irreversible damage. If the life control centers within the brain stem cease to function, the patient will die. This process of brain stem compression is called herniation (Figure 3-3), which is a neurosurgical emergency. The brain stem is very vulnerable and once compressed can be irrevocably damaged. Brain stem compression is almost invariably fatal since it causes destruction of the respiratory and other vital brain stem nuclei, leaving the patient comatose and completely dependent on the ventilator.

It is important to remember that any of the different types of brain injury can lead to herniation. Swelling, contusions, and bleeding can all lead to an increase in the amount of "stuff" inside the skull. To make room, the brain compresses, causing severe damage to important areas of the brain and brain stem. Herniation can sometimes be prevented by the administration of **mannitol, hyperventilation,** or surgery. There may be times, however, when the brain injury is so severe that all attempts to prevent herniation are futile.

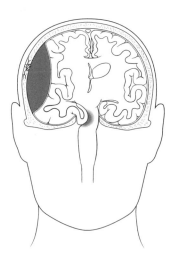

Figure 3-3 Herniation occurs when the brain compresses the brain stem. This can be secondary to different types of head injuries. This illustration depicts a skull fracture that has caused an epidural hematoma. The adjacent brain is "pushed aside" forcing the temporal lobe to compress the brain stem, causing damage.

INJURIES TO BLOOD VESSELS
Epidural Hematoma

This type of hemorrhage occurs from damage to one of the arteries that lie between the skull and the **dura.** Patients may develop an **epidural hematoma** after a minor, even negligible, head injury. Often there is a small fracture in the skull that tears an artery in the dura. Blood from the torn artery rapidly accumulates under the skull and pushes on the brain (Figure 3-4). Initially the patients may only have a brief loss of unconsciousness and then appear fine. However, as the mass of blood grows larger, it begins to compress the brain. The patient then becomes very sleepy, which can progress to unconsciousness as the expanding blood clot pushes on the normal brain. If the bleeding from the torn artery is not stopped with surgery, the brain compression can continue and lead to herniation. An epidural hematoma is typically considered a life-threatening condition, especially a large one, which is treated with emergency surgery.

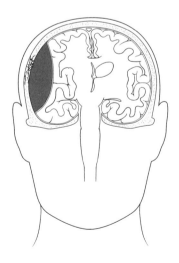

Figure 3-4 An epidural hematoma is usually secondary to a skull fracture that lacerates an artery in the dura. Blood rapidly accumulates between the skull and dura (giving it its classic convex shape), compressing the brain underneath.

Subdural Hematoma

This type of hemorrhage results from tears in the veins that lie on the surface of the brain. The force required to cause a **subdural hematoma** is usually greater than that needed to cause an epidural hematoma. Therefore, a subdural hematoma is often associated with other brain injuries, such as contusions, shearing, and lacerations. Unlike patients with an epidural hematoma, patients with a subdural hematoma usually are unconscious right after the injury because the blood is directly from injured brain rather than from an artery outside the brain (Figure 3-5). Patients with a subdural hematoma usually do not do as well as those with an epidural hematoma for this reason. They may or may not require surgery as the amount of blood may be too small to cause any brain compression.

Subarachnoid Hemorrhage

This kind of hemorrhage results from tears in the small blood vessels lying on or within the brain. Unlike a subdural hematoma, this condition usually does not result in a large accumulation of blood clot. **Subarachnoid hemorrhage** is fairly common and may be seen

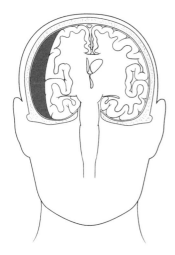

Figure 3-5 Subdural hematomas occur when the brain itself is damaged or when the veins between the brain and the skull are torn. The blood slowly accumulates on the surface of the brain (underneath the dura) and compresses the adjacent tissue. Cerebral contusions often accompany these injuries.

in minor or major head injuries. It is generally not life-threatening, but occasionally can cause delayed problems. As previously described, the brain contains cavities (i.e., ventricles) that are filled with clear CSF. This fluid is made within the ventricles and flows out of the brain. It then percolates over the top of the brain until it completely surrounds the brain and spinal cord. This fluid is constantly being made and reabsorbed by the body at an equivalent rate so that the total amount is always the same.

Subarachnoid blood may interfere with reabsorption of CSF by clogging up the specialized structures that drain off the fluid. This is analogous to leaves clogging a sewer grate. This accumulation of fluid is called **hydrocephalus** or "water on the brain" and may require surgical correction by insertion of a **ventriculoperitoneal shunt.** This complication is often not evident until days or weeks after the initial injury because it takes time for all the drains to become clogged. Hydrocephalus can also occur when there is a blood clot within the ventricles (Figure 3-6).

Subarachnoid hemorrhage can also lead to a condition called **vasospasm.** The blood, once it has escaped from the blood vessels, can irritate the smaller cerebral arteries which then go into spasm. The inside of the vasospastic arteries gets very small as the vessels squeeze in on themselves. As this process continues, the **lumen**

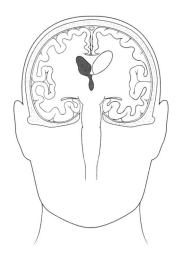

Figure 3-6 Intraventricular hemorrhage. Some injuries cause bleeding within the ventricles. The subsequent blood clot can "clog" the ventricular system, creating hydrocephalus. Placement of a ventriculostomy is often required in these instances to externally drain the CSF.

may completely close off. As blood is no longer able to flow through these vessels in spasm, the areas of the brain that these cerebral arteries were supplying with blood no longer receive the necessary oxygen. The brain cells begin to die, leading to further damage and strokes.

CEREBROSPINAL FLUID LEAK

As described earlier, the CSF is made within the ventricles. CSF drains out of the brain through internal channels, much like the pipes that run through our homes. In specific areas of the brain holes allow the fluid to percolate over the top of the brain. This results in the brain being surrounded by CSF on the inside and outside. This is similar to a water balloon immersed in a bucket of water.

The skull is commonly fractured in head injury. These fractures can occur on the **convexity of the skull** or at the base of the skull (Figure 3-7). The skull base is a platform of bone on which the brain rests. The convexity of the skull is the dome of bone that sits on top of the skull base. When either of these areas of bone is fractured, CSF can leak out through the hole. The resultant CSF leak

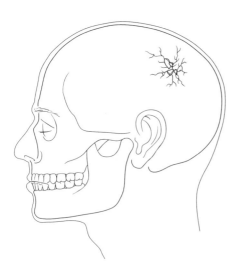

Figure 3-7 A skull fracture is commonly seen in head injuries. A skull fracture can be linear or convoluted. Sharp bone fragments can tear the underlying dura and result in a CSF leak.

increases the risk of the patient developing an infection in the brain called **meningitis.** While the hole in the skull gives the CSF a way out, it also provides a path for bacteria on the skin or in the nasal sinuses to get inside the brain. The meningitis caused by the bacteria can be a serious, life-threatening infection, which, in a severely injured patient, can lessen the chances for a good recovery.

Unfortunately, CSF leaks are not always easy to recognize. Fractures to the base of the skull tend to cause fluid leakage that travels down the back of the throat or into the sinuses, two areas that are not easily visualized. The good news is that about 95% of these situations stop on their own as the patient's body seals up the hole. Occasionally it persists and requires sophisticated radiologic scans to pinpoint the location of the abnormal pathway, enabling a surgeon to operate and close the hole.

GRADING HEAD INJURY

When a patient with head injury is taken to an emergency department, his or her neurologic status is evaluated to determine the severity of the injury. To accomplish this, a grading system, termed the **Glasgow Coma Scale** or **GCS,** has been developed. It is a simple and repeatable way to gain an understanding of the severity of a patient's neurologic injury. The GCS may also be used to predict the patient's chance for recovery. The scale ranges from 3 to 15, in which 3 is the worst case and 15 is a patient with normal to near-normal neurologic function. The health care team tests three response areas: motor, verbal, and eye. Under each category, varying degrees of response are each assigned a numerical value:

Motor Response (M)	Verbal Response (V)	Eye Opening (E)
6 Follows commands	5 Oriented	4 Spontaneous
5 Localizes pain	4 Confused	3 To voice
4 Withdraws from pain	3 Inappropriate	2 To pain
3 Decorticate posture	2 Gibberish	1 None
2 Decerebrate posture	1 None	
1 None		

Each of these categories is tested upon the initial examination of the patient and response values are added to give the patient a GCS score. This system is very valuable because it gives the physician a quick and easy way to get an initial sense of the seriousness of the patient's brain injury. The GCS is easy to do and can be done in just a few minutes, so it does not delay treatment. In addition to providing an efficient and reliable method of assessing the severity of the injury, the GCS has also been used to predict the patient's overall prognosis. With this in mind, it is important to realize that a patient's GCS score may be artificially lowered if the patient has been using drugs, alcohol, or if body temperature is too low. It also can be affected by injuries to the eyes, mouth, or spinal cord in which the patient loses the ability to respond verbally, open the eyes, or move. In the absence of these confounding factors, the GCS is a reliable way to assess the severity of a head injury.

Glasgow Coma Scale Scores

Severe Head Injury	GCS 3-8
Moderate Head Injury	GCS 9-11
Mild Head Injury	GCS 12-15

The GCS evaluation is repeated regularly while the patient is at the hospital. This enables the health care staff to consistently follow the patient's neurologic course. A sudden drop in the GCS score alerts the health care staff that something untoward may be happening that requires intervention. An increase in the GCS may indicate that the effects of drugs or alcohol are beginning to wear off or that the patient is improving.

BRAIN DEATH

Sometimes patients are so severely injured that they show no signs of brain function. When a patient is in this condition the question of brain death arises. **Brain death** is a clinical diagnosis that signifies the absence of any remaining brain function. The physician performs a detailed neurologic assessment that tests each component of the central nervous system to ensure that there is no residual brain function. Any sign of brain function rules out the existence of brain death. The brain death examination checks the cerebral cortex, midbrain, pons, and medulla for any signs of function. There are six specific tests that comprise the brain death examination. The results of these tests will tell the physician whether any or no part of the brain is functioning.

The physician shines a flashlight in the patient's eyes to check for pupillary response to light. If the pupils do not constrict in the bright light, this is a sign of midbrain death. The next test is application of a painful stimulus such as heavy pressure on the chest wall. If the patient does not respond to this stimulus, it indicates death of the cerebral cortex. Cold water is then placed in the patient's ear canal. Normally, there are characteristic eye movements as a result of this maneuver. If the patient's eyes remain fixed, this indicates death to part of the brain stem.

A tongue depressor is then applied to the back of the patient's throat to check for a **gag reflex.** If the patient does not cough or gag, this is a sign of brain stem death. Next, a cotton swab is applied to the patient's eye to see if the patient blinks. The normal response is involuntary blinking of both eyes. If the eyes fail to blink, destruction of the pons is verified. The last component is the apnea test. The patient is taken off the ventilator for a brief period of time to see if he or she is able to take a breath without the aid of the machine. If the patient does not breathe in five minutes, it is a sign that the respiratory centers in the brain stem are dead. If *all* six of these signs are present, the patient is considered brain dead.

Before performing a brain death examination the patient undergoes screening to ensure that there are no medicines or drugs in the system that would mimic brain death. Also, the patient's body temperature must be at least 95° F, as anything lower could conceal residual brain function. Once it has been proven that there are no drugs or medicines in the patient's system that could mimic brain death, and the proper body temperature is present, a formal brain death examination is performed.

One important concept to understand is that heart function is *not* a sign of brain function. Thus a person can be brain dead and still have a beating heart. The heart is made up of specialized cells that have their own internal pacemaker. In fact, the heart can be surgically removed from the body and continue to beat for several minutes on its own. So the presence of a beating heart does not exclude a diagnosis of brain death.

⚜ COMMONLY ASKED QUESTIONS ⚜

Is the patient considered to be in a coma?

Coma is a term used more by the public than the medical profession. While the GCS is used to assess the severity of head injury present, the term "coma" itself represents a general state of being unconscious. Therefore, anyone who is unconscious for a prolonged period is in a state of coma. However, the term suggests some notion of the amount of time that the patient will be unconscious, something that really cannot be accurately predicted or known. There are actually different degrees or phases of unconsciousness, and a patient can be improving although still unconscious.

What is the difference between an open head injury and a closed head injury? Which one is more severe?

Head injuries fall into two general types: open and closed. Both can occur in various types of traumatic accidents in which a particular force is delivered to the patient's head. An injury in which the brain and the dura can be seen through the wound is called an open head injury. The skull is typically fractured with the overlying skin lacerated (i.e., torn open) thus exposing the underlying dura and possibly the brain (if the dura is also torn). These types of injuries usually result when an object hits the head with a considerable force. Examples include hitting the windshield in an automobile accident, being hit in the head with a baseball bat, or falling prey to a gunshot to the head. Due to the large forces necessary to extensively fracture the skull, there is commonly significant brain damage at the site of impact in open head injuries. Surgery is usually required to debride (i.e., clean) the wounds in an attempt to prevent infection. Any bone fragments that were driven into the brain are removed, the skull fractures repaired as necessary, and the skin closed. The dura is also closed during the operation.

Closed head injuries describe those in which the brain remains covered by an intact skull. Despite the lack of a large hole in the skull and overlying skin, these injuries can also involve significant brain damage. In fact, the damage sustained in these types of injuries is commonly more diffuse. It is for this reason that closed head injuries tend to be more severe than open head injuries in terms of the amount of damage produced. Unlike open head injuries, in which there can be extensive damage at the site of impact, the diffuse brain injury that occurs in closed head injuries is not confined to one portion of the brain. The damage can occur throughout the brain and include the brain stem as well. Patients with severe closed head injuries are deeply unconscious and commonly have elevated ICPs. The elevated ICP can cause further damage as the brain swells and pushes up against the intact skull. Surgery is generally only indicated if there is a focal blood clot or contusion that requires removal.

What is hydrocephalus?

Hydrocephalus or "water on the brain" is a situation where the internal plumbing of the brain gets clogged up and no longer functions properly. The brain and spinal cord are bathed in CSF, which is continually made within the fluid-filled spaces inside the brain called ventricles. Normally, after circulating around the brain, this fluid drains out of the ventricles. Eventually the CSF is reabsorbed into the blood. Anything that blocks the normal flow of the CSF can lead to a build-up of fluid inside these fluid-filled spaces. As the fluid builds up within the ventricles, they begin to enlarge, much the way a balloon enlarges when it is filled with water. The pressure inside the brain (ICP) begins to increase as the CSF builds up within the ventricles. This increased pressure, if it gets too high, can cause damage to the brain by impeding the blood flow to the brain from the heart.

A common cause of hydrocephalus in head injury patients is

secondary to blood within the brain, particularly inside the ventricles. The blood, after it escapes from the blood vessels injured by the trauma, forms a clot that can act as a plug that blocks the ventricles. This can result in hydrocephalus and increased pressure within the brain. Sometimes this situation is only temporary and can be treated by placing a **catheter** into the fluid-filled spaces of the brain. This procedure is called a **ventriculostomy,** which allows direct drainage of the ventricles into a bag that hangs next to the patient. In some cases the blood clot is slowly dissolved by the brain and the blockage of the ventricles disappears, enabling the normal flow of CSF out of the brain. If this occurs, the ventriculostomy is usually no longer needed and is removed. In other situations, even though the blood clot dissolves, the drainage system remains blocked up and the normal CSF flow pathway remains nonfunctional. In these cases the patient requires constant drainage of the ventricles to prevent hydrocephalus and secondary increased pressure within the brain.

Due to concerns of infection and the impracticality of having a catheter protruding from the head permanently, these patients typically require a ventriculoperitoneal shunt. This procedure is performed in the operating room. A catheter is again placed into the ventricles, but rather than having it connected to a collection bag outside of the patient, it is connected to a second longer catheter that is tunneled beneath the skin and placed into the abdomen. Usually a valve is a component of this system, which allows drainage of the ventricles only when the pressure inside the brain is too high. Thus the ventriculoperitoneal shunt takes over for the natural drainage of the ventricles, draining the CSF internally into the abdomen only when needed.

Can you explain the GCS?

The GCS is a method to describe the severity of head injury based on the physical examination. This method was developed to provide uniformity in describing a patient's neurologic examination at any given time. The neurologic examination is a very important test used to assess how the patient's brain is doing after injury. By providing a standardized, uniform way of testing and describing the patient's examination findings, different members of the health care staff can consistently follow the patient's status. A decline in the GCS over time may suggest that some new process, such as a new hemorrhage or increased swelling, is occurring within the brain, raising the red flag that further investigation (typically a CT scan) is needed to find the problem.

The GCS is based on the patient's movements (motor response), whether the patient is talking and making sense (verbal response), and whether the patient opens his or her eyes (eye response). Each of these three categories has different ways the patient may respond, with each response graded (i.e., given a number). The higher the number, the more appropriate the response, and the lower the number, the worse the patient's neurologic condition. The numbers from each category's responses are then added together. The GCS is the sum of these three numbers and can range from 3 to 15. A GCS of 3 describes a patient who has no response at all, while a GCS of 15 indicates that a patient is neurologically normal.

In addition to providing a consistent method of following these patients neurologically (i.e., how well the brain is functioning), the GCS is also one factor used to predict the outcome of a patient with brain injury. Patients with a GCS of 3 to 8 are said to have severe head injury, those with a GCS of 9 to 11 have moderate head injury, and those with a GCS of 12 to 15 have mild head injury. In general, the lower the GCS, the less likely the patient will have a good outcome (i.e., these patients have a poor prognosis). As the GCS increases, the likelihood for a better outcome also increases. Although there are other factors, such as age and type of injury, on the whole patients with severe head injury do the worst, patients with mild head injury do the best, and patients with moderate head injury are in between.

Can a cervical injury cause brain damage?

Isolated cervical injuries, when severe, typically result in cervical spinal cord injury but not necessarily brain injury. These patients, however, can have many of the same signs as those with brain injury, such as differing degrees of paralysis. The problem is that, while cervical injury does not directly cause brain injury itself, the forces involved in the accident that led to the cervical injury were also imparted to the brain. Therefore, it is not uncommon to have both cervical and brain injuries in very serious accidents.

There are two specific instances where cervical injuries can lead to brain damage. One is any cervical injury, usually high in the cervical spinal cord, that stops the patient from breathing at the scene of the accident. If this period of time, in which no oxygen is being supplied to the brain, is longer than 4 minutes, brain damage can begin to occur. Longer periods of time without oxygen result in more extensive damage to the brain. Brain death is a possibility if the patient does not breathe for an extended period of time. The second situation in which a cervical injury can lead to brain damage is much more uncommon. The blood supply to the brain, which carries oxygen, is provided by two sets of arteries that run up through the neck. One set, called the **vertebral arteries,** actually run through the cervical neck bones that protect the spinal cord. Injuries that produce fractures in these bones can tear one or both of these arteries. This can produce a stroke in the brain or brain stem because the blood supply to these structures can be interrupted by tears in these vessels. The same is true for the **carotid arteries,** which do not run through the cervical neck bones but can be torn in serious cervical injuries.

Is the patient still considered to be in a coma if he or she is moving the arms and legs?

The term "coma" can be generally described as a state of prolonged unconsciousness. Patients with head injury can be unconscious but exhibit different actions. Some patients do not move at all while others are very active and appear agitated. There are actually several degrees of coma, which is partly why the GCS was developed. Two patients may both be unconscious but have vastly different degrees of injury to the brain. This is why the term "coma" is not used by the medical profession; the term is too vague to accurately describe the actual condition of the patient.

Patients in the different states of unconsciousness can exhibit different actions and responses to stimuli. Patients in a deep coma may not move at all, even to a painful stimulus, which is a bad sign and indicates that severe damage has occurred to the brain and/or the brain stem. Patients who do not show any response to stimuli, in the absence of any drugs or medications, very often do very poorly. Patients who move the arms and/or legs, while they still may be in a coma, have a much better chance for recovery. In general, the more movement the better. Patients tend to move more and show signs of purposeful movement (i.e., movements directed at achieving a particular goal) as they recover.

What is a lesion on the brain?

The word "lesion" is a catchall term that refers to any abnormal area within the brain. A lesion can be a hemorrhage, contusion, tumor, stroke, or abscess. Generally, it is used by physicians to describe the abnormality's location in the brain, such as "the lesion is in the patient's left internal capsule resulting in a right-sided hemiplegia." Two patients may have different lesions (one a tumor and the other a contusion) located in the same area of the brain. The resulting neurologic deficit will most likely be the same in each patient even though the respective problems are much different. The word "lesion" is essential jargon used by physicians to simplify communication between them. Unfortunately, the use of a single word to describe different things can be confusing to the layperson. If confronted with this term, or any other that increases confusion, simply ask the physician for a clearer explanation. Many times physicians do not realize they are adding to the confusion because they are so accustomed to using these terms. Remember that communication is a two-way street and open communication between the patient's family and the medical staff is crucial in obtaining proper care for the patient.

How much brain damage has been done?

In general, it helps to think of the damage caused by head injury as occuring in two phases: the "initial" and the "secondary." The initial injury occurs at the time of the accident as a result of the impact. This can result in contusions (bruises in the brain), bleeding, and the development of a blood clot, or shear injury, where the multiple connections within the brain are torn apart from the force of impact. The brain then reacts to these various forms of injury, usually by swelling. This is the secondary phase of damage. This swelling can push against portions of the brain that were initially not injured at the time of the accident, causing further injury, or it can produce elevated pressure throughout the brain, called elevated ICP. This can decrease the amount of blood that reaches the brain, which can cause further injury to both the damaged and nondamaged portions of the brain and brain stem. Both initial and secondary damage can cause brain cells to die and produce loss of function. Ultimately, it is the preservation of function that is the aim of all the medical treatment of head injury patients.

To assess the amount of initial damage, patients are given a neurologic examination when they arrive in the emergency department. This examination is basically the determination of their GCS, which includes the patient's movement response to stimuli (whether the patient moves spontaneously, only with stimuli, or exhibits automatic posturing movements), whether the patient can talk or not, and the patient's eye responses (whether the patient opens the eyes to various stimuli). A CT scan of the brain is usually also obtained in the emergency department to investigate what the brain looks like. Areas of contusion, swelling, fractures, and blood clots can typically be seen on the images produced by the CT scan. The combined information from the neurologic examination and the CT scan is then used to determine how much damage has taken place as a result of the injury.

Patients with brain injuries who can be helped with surgery are taken emergently to the operating room. Patients with nonsurgical injuries and those who have had surgery are then admitted to the

ICU for close medical attention. In general, the less the patient moves, talks, and opens the eyes, the worse the injury. Similarly, contusions and blood clots that are larger or multiple, or evidence of significant swelling, suggest more severe damage. However, in the brain and brain stem it is not always the amount of injury but the *location* of the injury that is important. Small areas of damage, if located in very important areas, such as the thalamus or brain stem, can lead to very serious injury and significant deficits. Larger areas of damage, although more extensive on the CT scan, may not produce as much deficit if located in portions of the brain that can tolerate more damage, such as the frontal and temporal lobes.

After the initial injury, the brain is very sensitive to any other insults or injury. Additional insults, such as low blood pressure, low oxygen levels, high body temperatures, and increased ICP, can cause further secondary damage. Therefore, secondary damage compounds the initial injury, making the total amount of damage more severe. This is a problem because patients with relatively small amounts of damage early on, as indicated by the initial neurologic examination and CT scan, may end up with significant damage as a result of this secondary injury process. It is this process that the health care staff attempts to counteract. As an analogy for this secondary injury process, falling from a bicycle may result in a small bruise on the knee but, by the second day after the seemingly small scrape, the knee is extremely swollen and tender. The same general process happens in the brain. Therefore, it can be difficult to ascertain just how much damage has occurred within the brain because the damage process may be continuing. That is why patients are watched so closely in the ICU, with frequent neurologic examinations and sometimes multiple CT scans.

Will the brain repair itself?

The brain is unique in that after a certain age no new brain cells are made. This is quite different from other organs, such as the liver or skin, where new cells are constantly being made. While a cut in the skin or a liver laceration can heal as new cells are made by these organs, such is not the case in the brain. **Neurons** (i.e., brain cells) that die are lost forever; new ones are not made to take their place. Hence, the brain cannot repair irreversibly damaged areas. Depending on the location of the damage, permanent functional loss can occur. Some patients may show some improvement, however, if the surrounding area can compensate for the lost function such that the healthy surrounding brain takes over control of the lost function. This capacity to compensate generally decreases with age.

It should be kept in mind, however, that not all injuries produce irreversible damage and neuronal death. Similarly, while irreversible damage may occur within a given area, the cells surrounding that area may have compromised function but not to the degree that it is irreversible. Therefore, the key in treating these patients is to save these borderline neurons from developing further damage and thus preserve as much function as possible.

Does the speed of the moving object have a direct correlation with the severity of the head injury?

Head injury is the result of a particular force imparted on the brain. In general, the more force applied to the brain during impact, the more damage occurs. There are other factors that also play a role in determining the severity of the resultant injury. These include the health of the patient's brain prior to the accident, whether there was a period of time in which no oxygen was being delivered to the brain after the accident, and the amount of time that elapsed between the accident and the initiation of treatment. All of these factors, including the force applied to the brain during the accident, act together to increase the severity of the head injury.

The speed of a moving object, such as a bullet fired from a gun, relates to this force. For example, high velocity bullets generally cause more damage as they move through tissue than lower velocity bullets. The same is true for motor vehicle accidents. Patients involved in high-speed accidents typically have more severe injuries than those traveling at slower speeds at the time of the accident. The same is true for head injuries as a result of a fall, where patients who fall from greater heights tend to have more severe injuries.

Therefore, there is a general relationship between the speed and force of the injury and the resultant severity, with additional factors also playing a role.

How much damage did the bullet cause?

The damage produced by a gunshot wound to the head is dependent on several different factors. An important distinction is whether the bullet actually penetrated the skull and entered the brain. Some gunshot wounds do not penetrate the skull. In these instances the bullet ricochets off the skull instead of penetrating it and entering the brain tissue. This type of injury can still cause significant damage to the brain but in general, these patients do better than those with penetrating gunshot wounds. Nonpenetrating gunshot wounds tend to be secondary to lower velocity bullets while high velocity bullets tend to penetrate the skull more often and produce considerably more damage. This illustrates the fact that a large portion of the brain damage that results from these injuries relates to the velocity of the bullet and not necessarily the size of the bullet. As the bullet travels through the brain, the energy and forces carried in the speeding bullet are quickly transferred to the brain tissue. This is somewhat analogous to a speed boat traveling through the water. The wake of force traveling behind the bullet spreads throughout the brain causing tremendous damage. The faster the bullet is moving, the larger the wake. Victims of such high velocity gunshot wounds to the head are usually devastated and have no evidence of brain or brain stem function (i.e., they are brain dead).

Another factor to be considered is the location of the bullet's path. Bullets that travel through one side of the brain and then cross over to the opposite side create tremendous damage. Patients commonly do not survive this type of injury. Bullets that penetrate the skull but do not pass through too much brain may only cause focal damage. Depending on the area injured, the patient may or may not have associated functional loss. In contrast, gunshot wounds that damage the brain stem are instantaneously fatal.

How can you tell the location of the entry and exit wounds?

The terms "entry" and "exit" are used to describe any gunshot wound. The entry wound is the location where the bullet enters the body and the exit wound is where it leaves the body. These are identified in an attempt to determine the direction the bullet was traveling and its path within the body. It can be a difficult task, however, to accurately identify the entry and the exit in a patient with two apparent gunshot wounds on the head. In addition, not all patients have exit wounds, but rather just an entry wound with the bullet remaining within the brain.

In general, entry wounds are smaller than exit wounds. This is because bullets tend to "tumble" after penetrating the skull. This tumbling action creates more and more damage as the bullet moves through the brain and creates extensive damage upon exiting the skull. CT scans can be used to help determine the path the bullet traveled within the brain. This information is then used to determine the location of the entry and exit wounds. While the exact determination of the entry and exit wounds is usually inconsequential to the devastated patient, such information is useful for the criminal investigation of the case.

What does "no gag, no corneals, no cough reflex" mean?

These terms refer to the absence of normal cranial reflexes. The brain stem controls some of our body's most basic automatic functions. These reflexive actions are performed without any conscious awareness. For example, when a physician sticks a tongue depressor deep into our throat, we gag even if we try not to gag. The brain stem recognizes the stimulus of something touching the back of the throat and instantly signals the muscles of the throat to contract. This gag reflex is an important defense mechanism. The act of gagging helps expel foreign material, such as food, that gets caught in our throats. The corneal and cough reflexes are similar in that they are automatic protective responses under direct control of the brain stem. The absence of these reflexes indicates serious damage to the brain stem. In fact, the corneal, gag and cough reflexes are all things that the physician checks when doing a brain death examination. The absence of all brain stem reflexes, which includes the gag, corneal, cough, and pupillary reflexes, in combination with no respiratory drive (patient does not breathe) and no response to any type of stimuli, is consistent with brain death.

What is the difference between a concussion and a contusion?

The basic difference is that a concussion is a symptom while a contusion describes a damaged area within the brain. Both can occur in head injuries. A concussion describes a situation where the patient briefly loses consciousness from a head injury. These patients regain consciousness within a few minutes and do not have any neurologic abnormalities (essentially the brain is momentarily stunned). CT scans of these patients do not show any abnormality. They may have transient headaches, amnesia, or slight personality changes in which they are drowsy, irritable, and confused. These symptoms usually resolve within a few days.

A contusion refers to a brain injury in which there is structural damage to the brain itself. This damage (which is essentially a bruise on the brain) can be seen on a CT scan as a focal area of abnormality. The clinical signs and symptoms may be identical to that of a contusion but more often the symptoms are more complex and last much longer. The patient often shows focal weakness or sensory loss that corresponds to the sight of the brain contusion. For example, a concussion may make a patient confused and have slurred speech but a contusion in the speech area of the brain may leave the patient unable to speak at all. Contusions tend to resolve over a period of days to weeks but the deficit they cause may improve but may never go away completely.

What causes lacerations in the brain and how do they cause damage? Can they be repaired?

Brain lacerations are usually the result of penetrating brain injuries. Any object that enters the cranial cavity can tear through the brain. Open head injuries in which the bony fragments of the skull are forcefully driven into the brain can cause severe tearing of brain and blood vessels. The damage that results is a direct reflection of the size, velocity, and entry site of the projectile. Generally, the bigger and faster the projectile, the more brain damage it will cause.

Repairing the damage is limited to removing areas of dead brain and hemorrhage, stopping bleeding from torn blood vessels, and reconstructing the dura and skull damaged by the projectile. Lacerating injuries of the brain are more severe in that they can lead to many secondary injuries not apparent at the time the patient arrives at the hospital. These secondary injuries can result from brain edema that develops over the days following injury or from stroke that is a consequence of vascular injury. Typically there is not much to repair surgically, rather the surgeon must remove dead and foreign tissue and clean the wound to prevent an infection from developing.

What is the cause of brain shearing?

Brain shearing describes the injury in which the neurons in the brain have been twisted or stretched by complex forces applied to the head. Remember, the brain is not a rigid structure, so it will move inside the skull in response to an applied force. When we are struck in the head, the head and brain turn away from the impact but not always in the same direction or at the same speed. This turning or twisting causes rotational forces to develop within the brain. These rotational forces are similar to the pressure applied to a washcloth when someone wrings out the water. The twisting causes incredible pressure on the nerve fibers in the brain and often leads to overwhelming loss of brain cells and their connections. This can lead to very extensive injuries to the deep structures of the brain, such as the **corpus callosum, pons,** and **midbrain.** These shearing-type injuries can be one of the more devastating injuries. Patients with this type of injury may be comatose indefinitely.

What causes the brain to swell?

After a head injury the brain responds to the damage produced by invoking the normal immunologic healing responses that occur in other places in our body. These healing responses are designed to bring cells and materials (proteins, vitamins, chemicals, etc.) to the area of injury. These materials are specially designed to help repair the damage, fight off infection, and stop bleeding. These chemicals also act on blood vessels in a certain way that makes them leaky. This helps these specialized cells get into the brain and enter the site of injury. This process is easily understood by anyone who has ever twisted an ankle. The swelling that occurs is the body trying to limit the extent of the damage and repair that which has already been injured. Essentially the same swelling process occurs within the brain.

The problem unique to the brain is that it is encased in a rigid structure. When all the special cells and material arrive, they increase the contents of the cranial cavity. This leads to increased ICP and thus leads to further injury. A vicious cycle can occur in which injury leads to swelling and swelling causes more injury, which again brings about more swelling, and so on.

How long will the edema continue to increase?

This depends on the severity of the initial injury and whether the patient responds to the treatments directed at decreasing the brain swelling. The problem is that when the brain swells it can cause more damage, which then results in more swelling, more damage, and so on. To be successful, the health care staff must break this cycle and get the swelling under control early. This is not always possible, however, especially in those patients who suffered extensive brain injury at the time of the accident. The crucial time for cerebral edema is about the first 7 to 10 days after the injury. If the ICP can be controlled (and enough blood can be supplied to the brain during that time), the cerebral edema usually begins to decrease after 7 to 10 days. The addition of any other damaging factors, such as brain infection, electrolyte abnormalities or poor oxygen content in the blood (secondary to lung problems), or the development of a stroke, can increase the damage to the brain. Any increase in the damage to the brain will result in further and prolonged swelling.

How long will it take for the edema to go away?

The injury that occurs at the time of the accident causing the brain to swell is termed cerebral edema. As the brain begins to swell in response to the injury, more damage can take place. While little can be done for the injury that results from the initial accident, it is this secondary damage process, caused by factors, including cerebral edema, that the health care staff attempts to minimize. Once the secondary damage is halted and the brain is provided a healthy environment in which to recover, the cerebral edema will start to go away. Thus the time it takes for the cerebral edema to go away is dependent on how long it takes to stop the secondary damage process, as well as the amount of cerebral edema that was present at that time. The more swelling, the more difficult it is to get under control, and the longer it will take to go away once it is controlled.

It is this race to control the secondary damage process, in which cerebral edema plays a role, that the health care staff is trying to win. The longer the secondary damage process is allowed to continue, the more damage occurs to the brain. More damage can result in more loss of function, which is ultimately what the health care staff is trying to preserve. Hopefully, once the process is controlled, no further damage will occur in the brain and it can then recover.

What can be done to decrease the ICP?

Elevated ICP is a common problem in head injury patients. As the ICP increases, it acts to impede the normal blood flow to the injured brain. This can result in further damage to the brain. Therefore, it is important to keep the ICP under control if at all possible. There are a variety of ways to help decrease the ICP. These methods include medications and surgical procedures. In general, less intense methods are used initially, with the more involved treatments reserved for those patients who do not respond. For example, one very simple maneuver that may help to decrease the ICP is to raise the head on the bed 30 degrees. Most patients with head injury have this done right away.

In order to measure the ICP, a ventriculostomy or **Camino intracranial monitor** is placed in the patient's brain. Camino monitors are placed in the surface of the brain and provide ICP measurements. Ventriculostomies are inserted into the ventricles. This is a more involved procedure as the catheter must be passed though the brain into the ventricles. It has the benefit, however, of not only measuring the ICP but also draining CSF from the ventricles. This can be a very valuable method to help control the ICP.

The ICP can build up not only from brain swelling but also from other areas of the body. Agitation, significant restlessness, repeated coughing or gagging, and "fighting the ventilator" (when the patient's own disordered breathing pattern acts against the ventilator's assistance) can all increase the ICP as measured by the Camino monitor or ventriculostomy. While the ICP displayed by the monitor is high, it is high because of these other "nonbrain" factors. To remove the effect of these body factors on the ICP, some patients may be given sedation and chemical paralytics. These act to calm agitated patients and remove any muscular activity that may be increasing the ICP. If the ICP was high because of these body factors it usually drops significantly with the administration of these medications.

Another medication that is usually very useful in controlling the ICP is mannitol. This acts to dry out the swollen brain by removing water from the brain tissue. The water is drawn out of the brain, put into the blood, and then urinated out by the body. The urinary output usually increases significantly after mannitol is given. However, care must be taken when administrating this medication because it can cause **electrolyte** abnormalities and kidney damage if too much is given. It is for these reasons that only a certain amount of mannitol can be given. Patients who do not respond to the above medications may be given **pentobarbital.** This medication, used as a last resort in patients who have high ICPs, places the patient in a deep chemical coma. Pentobarbital may help to protect the brain until the swelling and ICP decrease. This can be effective in controlling the ICP in some patients.

There are also surgical procedures that can be performed to help control the ICP. Any patient with elevated ICP caused by a large blood clot or contusion is taken to the operating room to have the abnormality removed. This can be very effective in controlling the ICP because it directly addresses the reason why the ICP was high. It is for this reason that patients with high ICPs have frequent CT scans. The CT scans are used to identify areas of damage that can be successfully treated surgically. Although there may not be a localized area of injury on the CT scan, some patients may benefit from having a **bone flap** removed. This procedure, in which a portion of the skull is removed and left out, may provide more space to accommodate the swollen brain. In some instances, portions of the brain may also be removed to further increase the space available for the swollen brain. These are obviously very aggressive measures to help control the ICP. Such procedures are more or less a last resort and the benefit to the patient may be minimal.

Is vessel injury common in head injuries?

There is a wide spectrum of head injury types, some of which involve injury to blood vessels, such as an epidural or subdural hematoma, and others, such as **hypoxic** injury, that cause brain damage without involving the blood vessels. However, some degree of blood vessel injury is commonly seen in head injuries. There are two types of vessels, arteries and veins. Arteries carry oxygenated blood to the brain under relatively high pressure. Veins carry the blood out of the brain after the oxygen has been extracted by the brain tissue. These vessels carry blood at a lower pressure than the arteries. Therefore, an injury to a large artery can quickly lead to a large amount of bleeding due to the relatively high pressure in these vessels, while vein injuries tend to bleed at a slower rate. Regardless of the type of vessel injured, the bleeding usually stops by itself after a certain point. It is relatively uncommon to lose a lot of blood from a bleeding vessel in the brain. The exception is in very small children and infants.

Although the bleeding usually stops, the resultant blood clot, if it is large enough, can compress the surrounding normal brain leading to further injury. Surgery may be necessary to remove the blood clot and decompress the brain. An epidural hematoma is an example of such an injury. This injury results from a tear in an artery, usually from a skull fracture, on the surface of the dura. Surgery is often performed to remove the blood clot and stop the artery from bleeding. Subdural hematomas can result from injury to the veins on the surface of the brain. These injuries also typically require surgery to remove the blood clot. Subarachnoid hemorrhage, an injury that usually does not require surgery, typically results from injury to the very small arteries on the surface of the brain. Again, the bleeding from these small arteries usually stops on its own. The same is true for the contusions (bruises within the brain tissue) that have some degree of blood loss associated with the damaged area.

How do other bodily injuries affect brain injuries?

The brain can be injured in any number of ways. These include direct impact or tearing of the actual brain tissue, any circumstance in which there is not enough oxygen supplied to the brain, conditions that decrease the blood's ability to form a clot, and anything that results in a brain infection. Any injury to the body that forces one of these situations can cause further brain damage.

Skull fractures in which portions of the bone are driven into the brain can directly tear the brain parenchyma. Extensive facial fractures, when they occur in the presence of frontal skull fractures, can also result in the same type of tearing injury to the brain. In addition to directly tearing the brain tissue, these injuries can also lead to CSF leaks and subsequent meningitis. Meningitis can also occur as a result of infections located elsewhere in the body. Bacteria can invade the blood from these infections and travel to the brain, resulting in meningitis.

Bodily injuries that result in decreased oxygen and blood supply to the brain can also cause further damage. These types of injuries are considered life-threatening and are treated immediately. Damage to the major internal organs, such as the heart, liver, and major arteries, can produce significant blood loss and this can cause low blood pressure. The brain, as well as the rest of the entire body, does not receive enough blood and oxygen in these situations. Severe injuries can also decrease the blood's ability to form blood clots. This can produce enlargement of blood collections within the brain as a result of the initial injury. While the blood pressure may be adequate, damage to the lungs can be such that the blood does not get enough oxygen. In these circumstances the brain receives enough blood but not enough oxygen, resulting in further brain damage. Lung injuries that lead to decreased oxygen content within the blood are also considered potentially life-threatening and are treated immediately.

CHAPTER
4

Lab Work and Imaging:
Understanding the Pictures
and Tests

I t is important to understand that the condition of head injury patients can change from moment to moment. The injury process does not stop at the time of the accident but can continue for several days. A vital aspect in the care of these patients is to quickly identify any changes in the patient's condition and intervene if necessary. By rapidly correcting any abnormalities, the chances improve for a better recovery. Part of this constant surveillance is a battery of tests and pictures that are used by the health care staff to assess the ever-changing status of the patient. These tests, which include blood work and x-ray films, can be instrumental in identifying a life-threatening condition or can be used to monitor how well a particular treatment is working. Some of the tests are routinely performed to constantly monitor the patient's status, while others are ordered only if something about the patient's condition suggests that further investigation is warranted. Following are general descriptions of some of the tests and "pictures" that may be ordered by the health care staff.

BLOOD GAS

Evaluating the blood gas, which is also called the **arterial blood gas** or **ABG,** is a laboratory test run on blood drawn from an artery. Arteries carry blood that is rich in oxygen while veins generally carry blood that already has the oxygen taken from it by the cells in the body. The blood for this test is usually drawn from the artery in the wrist (where you can feel a pulse). Typically, patients already have an **arterial line** (the catheter in the wrist or groin that constantly monitors the blood pressure) from which the arterial blood for this test can be drawn. This is convenient because the patient does not need to be stuck with a needle every time the test is performed.

In general, the ABG measures how well the patient is breathing, either on the **ventilator** (breathing machine) or without assistance. Specifically, the amount of oxygen, carbon dioxide (the gas which is exhaled with every breath), and the relative acidity in the blood is measured. The determination of the oxygen content is used to adjust the amount of oxygen that the patient is receiving. If the value is too low, which is dangerous to the patient and the injured brain, more oxygen is given. Low values may suggest that the patient has a problem in the lungs, such as undiagnosed **pneumonia.** It may also indicate that the patient is not breathing well enough without assistance and may need to be **intubated** (a breathing tube inserted to help out with breathing). When the oxygen values are high, less oxygen is given since too much oxygen can actually damage the lung, causing it to get firm, which eventually decreases the ability of oxygen to enter the blood.

The blood gas test also measures the amount of carbon dioxide in the blood. During normal breathing, oxygen is inhaled into the lungs and carbon dioxide is exhaled. The amount of carbon dioxide in the blood is generally dependent on the ventilation rate (how fast the breathing is). The faster the breathing, the more carbon dioxide is exhaled and, hence, the lower the carbon dioxide content will be in the blood. Patients who are agitated and breathing very fast exhibit low carbon dioxide levels on the ABG test. Some patients with elevated **intracranial pressures** or **ICPs** (from brain swelling) and who are on the ventilator will be made to breathe fast on purpose. This is called **hyperventilation,** which can temporarily decrease the ICP. The carbon dioxide content in the blood gas test is used by the health care staff to determine if the patient is being hyperventilated enough (i.e., the carbon dioxide level is low enough) or whether the patient is being hyperventilated too much (i.e., the carbon dioxide level is too low), in which case the breathing rate is turned down on the ventilator. In addition, patients who are not on the ventilator can be monitored with serial blood gases to make sure that they are breathing adequately.

If the carbon dioxide level gets too high, which can increase the pressure in the injured brain, it suggests that the patient is having problems breathing adequately and may need to be intubated. Conversely, patients who are on the ventilator but appear to be doing well enough to have the breathing tube removed **(extubated)** can be assessed using the ABG measurements as well. Normal oxygen and carbon dioxide values on the ABG test indicate that the patient may be breathing well enough and that the breathing tube and machine are no longer necessary. Overall, the ABG test is very valuable in monitoring the vital aspects of the patient's condition and treatment.

ELECTROLYTES

Evaluating **electrolytes** is another blood test, but one in which blood is drawn from the vein rather than the artery. There are various components to this particular test but, in general, it measures the content of different electrolytes that are normally found in the blood. These electrolytes include sodium, potassium, chloride, bicarbonate, urea nitrogen, and creatinine. The levels of these electrolytes are used to assess various aspects of the patient's condition. As with the other tests, when an abnormality is identified, steps can be taken to correct it.

Sodium, a component of salt, is a very important electrolyte used by the body for many different functions. The **nervous sys-**

tem, which includes the brain, relies heavily on sodium to function properly. The sodium level is also an indirect measurement of the amount of water in the body. This is a vital part in the care of head injury patients, especially those with severe head injury since it involves the management of water (or fluid content) within the brain and body. The amount of fluid within the blood needs to be high enough to ensure that systemic blood pressure is at an adequate level to get oxygen into the brain. If the fluid status of the patient is too low, it may be difficult to keep the systemic blood pressure high enough to get the blood, and hence the oxygen, into the brain. On the other hand, too much fluid in the blood may lead to brain swelling and increased ICP, which in turn can cause damage to the already injured brain. The sodium level obtained from the electrolyte blood test is one measurement that is used to answer these fluid status questions.

Head injury itself can also affect the fluid status and sodium levels. Centers within the brain play a role in the control of fluid status. If these centers are damaged from the head injury, abnormal alterations in the body's fluid control mechanisms can occur. This can result in the body holding on to too much water by essentially turning off the kidneys, a condition called **syndrome of inappropriate antidiuretic hormone** or **SIADH.** This condition results in too much water being retained by the body. The body may become bloated and the brain can swell, causing elevated ICPs. The elevated ICP can lead to less blood getting to the brain. When SIADH occurs, the sodium levels get very low, which can cause **seizures** in the patient. The treatment for SIADH is to *reduce* the amount of fluids given to the patient.

The opposite situation can also occur with head injury. Instead of retaining too much water, the kidneys may release too much water, a condition called **diabetes insipidus.** (This has no relation to the diabetes where the sugar levels are too high.) In this condition the injured brain sends the wrong signal to the kidneys and the patient urinates almost constantly. The fluid status gets too low, which can decrease the blood pressure. Low blood pressure can lead to inadequate blood supply to the brain. When the sodium levels get very high (the opposite of SIADH), the treatment is to give a lot of fluid to the patient to make up for what is being lost by the kidneys. Sometimes it may be necessary to give a medication called **desmopressin acetate** or **DDAVP,** which may correct the problem.

Another blood measurement, called the **serum osmolarity,** measures the concentration of the blood and is used in conjunction with the serum sodium levels. The values for these are also useful when patients are receiving **mannitol.** Mannitol is a medication that helps decrease the swelling in the brain. As with many things, however, too much of a good thing may be harmful. Mannitol can cause kidney damage if too much is given. The serum sodium and osmolarity tests are used to assess whether it is safe to give additional doses of mannitol.

The other electrolytes routinely checked are potassium, creatinine, and blood urea nitrogen. Potassium is important for proper nervous system and heart function. Patients with pre-existing heart problems, especially those with abnormal heart rhythms, as well as patients who sustain injury to the heart from the accident, are very sensitive to the serum potassium levels. Levels that are too high or too low may cause abnormal heart rhythms, which can be fatal. Therefore, the serum potassium level is watched very carefully and corrected when necessary. Serum creatinine and blood urea nitrogen are indicators of how the kidneys are functioning. Careful attention is placed on these values if the patient is suspected of having kidney damage or is receiving mannitol.

X-RAY FILMS

Included in the constant surveillance of head injury patients are a variety of x-ray films. These pictures are particularly useful when looking at the lungs and bones. Chest x-ray films are routinely taken to make sure that the lungs are inflated properly and to check for any evidence of pneumonia. If one of the lungs appears deflated (called a **pneumothorax**) a chest tube may be placed into the chest cavity to reinflate the lung. Antibiotics can be given if there is evidence of pneumonia. These pictures can also be used to make sure that the breathing tube is in the correct location in those patients who have one in place, as well as to make sure that any intravenous lines placed in the large veins in the neck are in the correct location. Blood, from lung damage, can also be seen on chest x-ray films.

X-ray films are also used in patients who may have a neck fracture. The bones in the neck can be evaluated to make sure that all the bones are in the proper position. The same is true for any other broken bone that may be present in the body. Depending on what the bones look like on the x-ray films, the health care staff may make adjustments to realign the bones into the proper position. Patients with feeding tubes or other tubes placed into the stomach might have x-ray films taken of the abdomen to make sure that the tubes are in the correct location. These same abdominal x-ray films can also be used to see if there is any build-up of air within the intestines, something that can occur if there is a blockage within the intestines or in patients who are paralyzed.

COMPUTED TOMOGRAPHY

Another type of x-ray, the **computed tomography** or **CT** scan (sometimes called the "cat scan") is instrumental in taking pictures of the brain, skull, and bones in the face. CT scans are very good at detecting blood within the brain and can be used to see if there is any swelling or compression of the brain. Most patients with head injury have a head CT scan when they arrive at the hospital. This helps to identify the extent of the brain injury and to see if there is any collection of blood that may require an operation. Some injuries may not show up immediately on this first CT scan, especially if it is taken very soon after the accident. Depending on the patient's condition and what was seen on the first CT scan, another one might be taken within the next 24 hours to be sure nothing has been missed, or to closely monitor a small collection of blood that was seen initially. Brand-new blood will show up white on the CT scan and if a large blood clot is seen, the patient may need emergency surgery. Patients who do not require surgery are typically taken to the intensive care unit or ICU, especially those with severe head injury, for close monitoring. If there is any change noted on any of the serial examinations performed by the health care staff, the patient is given another CT scan. This is to ensure that the change is not due to something that may be corrected with emergency surgery, such as a new or enlarging blood clot.

CT scans are also used to check the size of the fluid-filled spaces within the brain called the **ventricles.** Blood can also be seen within these deep structures, as can size. Some patients develop a blockage in this internal plumbing system that results in a build-up of fluid. The ventricles become enlarged and can cause increased pressure within the brain. This is called **hydrocephalus,** which can be easily seen on the CT scan. The fluid build-up can be treated by inserting a catheter (a **ventriculostomy**) into the dilated ventricles to drain the excess fluid. Sometimes this remains a permanent problem, in which case the patient needs a **ventriculoperitoneal shunt.** The position of the ventricles is also checked on the CT scan. These paired, fluid-filled structures are normally located symmetrically in the center of the brain.

Anything causing compression on one side of the brain, such as a blood clot or localized swelling in one of the lobes of the brain, will cause the ventricles to be pushed over to the other side. The spaces around the brain stem, in which the life control center is located, can also be checked. A large amount of swelling and high pressure within the brain can cause the brain to push against this very important structure. This can injure the brain stem, causing significant damage and even death. The CT scan is a very good method for determining just how much space is around the brain stem. In situations where the CT scan shows very little space around this life control center, the health care staff may initiate more intense measures to keep the brain swelling down.

In addition to looking at the brain, the CT scan is also used to evaluate the bone in the skull and face. Head injury patients often have associated fractures in the face and skull. Although skull fractures usually heal on their own without surgery, many facial fractures will not heal correctly unless treated surgically. The CT scan can locate any facial fractures that may be present. Depending on the configuration and extent of these facial fractures, surgery may or may not be necessary.

MAGNETIC RESONANCE IMAGING

Magnetic resonance imaging or **MRI** is another method to take pictures of the brain. This method uses a very large magnet instead of the x-ray beams used in CT scans. The MRI study produces much more detailed images of the brain and brain stem. This is of particular benefit in looking at the brain stem, a structure that is not seen very well on CT scans. Areas of injury to the brain stem can be seen on the MRI study if they are old enough. While little can be done for these areas of brain stem injury, MRI is used to determine the likely outcome for the patient. Such a determination is made based on the location and the extent of the injury. CT scans are used more frequently than MRI because the information obtained from the CT scan may be used to intervene on the patient's behalf (i.e., surgery or more aggressive treatment). MRI studies also take much longer than CT scans, and it may not be safe to have patients with severe head injury in the MRI scanner for a long period of time. Additionally, no metal objects can be brought into the MRI scanner because it uses such a powerful magnet. Many of the monitors and some of the catheters used to treat these patients have metallic parts, which excludes the use of MRI.

TRANSCRANIAL DOPPLER AND ANGIOGRAPHY

Some patients sustain vascular injury as a component of the head injury. Various different vascular injuries have been seen in patients with head injury, ranging from large tears in the major vessels within the neck and brain, to relatively small areas of damage to the vessels. Such vascular injuries can cause additional damage to the brain by depriving necessary oxygen to areas within the brain. In addition, the blood itself, which escaped outside of the blood vessels as a result of the injury, can lead to significant irritation of the noninjured blood vessels. This irritation can produce **vasospasm,** which in turn can lead to decreased blood and oxygen delivery to the normal areas of brain tissue. Prolonged periods of oxygen deprivation to the brain can lead to brain cell death and strokes.

In an attempt to assess whether the patient's brain is receiving enough blood, the **transcranial Doppler** may be used. This device uses sound waves to measure how fast the blood is flowing in the various blood vessels within the neck and brain. This device is similar to the ultrasound devices used to visualize a fetus prior to birth. By determining the speed that the blood is flowing within the blood vessels, the health care team can get an estimation as to whether any vasospasm is present. This device can also help determine if there is any blood flow in a given vessel in patients if there is a concern as to whether the injury interrupted the normal blood flow in a particular vessel. The benefit of this test is that it can be performed at the bedside without having to move the patient to another location. The drawback is that it can be somewhat inaccurate in actually determining if vasospasm is present. There is also a certain amount of subjectivity involved such that the vessels are not actually visualized.

In patients in whom vasospasm is suspected or when better visualization of the vascular anatomy is necessary, angiography is performed. An **angiogram** is a picture (i.e., an x-ray film) that displays the cerebral vascular anatomy. This allows the health care team to directly visualize all the different vessels (i.e., arteries and veins) within the neck and brain. This is made possible through the administration of dye into the arteries, followed by a series of x-ray films taken quickly in succession. A catheter is typically placed into the artery in the groin. Another catheter is threaded up this artery, back through the major arteries in the body, and finally into the major arteries of the brain. In addition to enabling visualization of the various cerebral vessels, various different interventions (i.e., treatments) can also be performed during this procedure. These include the administration of drugs to reverse vasospasm, manually reopen closed-down blood vessels with a balloon, and insert very small metal coils or balloons to occlude leaks in the blood vessels or abnormalities in the blood vessel wall. This procedure, unlike transcranial Doppler, must be performed in a special room.

EEG

An electroencephalogram or **EEG** records the electrical activity within the brain. This is done by placing multiple small metal disks called "electrodes" on the patient's scalp. Each electrode is connected to a small wire that is then connected to the EEG recording machine. This machine records the electrical activity in different areas within the brain. The recordings, which are a collection of multiple spikes and waves, are either printed on a continuously running piece of paper or displayed on a computer screen. The health care team can use this information to identify any electrical abnormalities such as a seizure within the brain. Most patients do not have seizures all the time, so it may be necessary to have an EEG continuously monitoring the electrical activity to determine if the patient is actually having seizures. This is called a "24-hour EEG." Continuous EEG monitoring may also be used in patients who are in **pentobarbital coma.** Although this brain wave test is good at identifying electrical seizure activity, it has little, if any, ability to predict the type of recovery the patient will have.

•———❧ COMMONLY ASKED QUESTIONS ❧———•

What information do you get from ABGs and how does it affect the brain?

The ABG, or arterial blood gas, is a laboratory test that measures various aspects of the blood. Included in this assay is the amount of oxygen and carbon dioxide contained within the blood. These are the gases that are put into and taken out of the blood by the lungs. Oxygen is necessary to keep cells within the body functioning properly and alive. Carbon dioxide is a waste product that is taken out of the blood and exhaled from the body by the lungs with every breath. Knowing how much oxygen is in the blood helps the health care staff determine whether enough oxygen is getting to the body and brain. Low oxygen levels on the ABG test indicate to the staff that more oxygen should be given to the patient. The combination of the oxygen and carbon dioxide levels on the ABG test also indicate how well the lungs are functioning. If the patient is on a ventilator, the settings can be changed to optimize the oxygen and carbon dioxide content within the blood if these values show as abnormal on the ABG test. Further, the carbon dioxide level is used to adjust the breathing rate of patients who are being hyperventilated (made to breathe fast on purpose) to help treat increased ICP.

Why do you monitor sodium levels and osmolarity?

Most patients with significant head injury have their blood serum and osmolarity measured. This is more important in patients who require the use of mannitol to control their ICP. Mannitol lowers ICP but it also acts to lower the amount of water in the circulating blood. Shortly after a patient is given mannitol, a large amount of dilute urine is usually passed. The urine is very light in color because it is mostly water. This is the water that was pulled out of the blood by the mannitol. The actual mechanism is more complex but, for the purposes of this discussion, think of mannitol as a magnet that draws water out of the blood. As water leaves the bloodstream, the blood becomes more concentrated. Think of a pot of coffee that has been left on the burner all day. At the end of the day, the water in the coffee has evaporated leaving behind a highly concentrated undrinkable liquid. The same thing happens to the blood when a patient is given mannitol. The sodium level and osmolarity measure just how concentrated the blood is. If the blood becomes too concentrated, the patient may develop kidney problems. The blood is filtered by the kidneys to make urine. Urine is essentially waste products that the body does not need and for this reason are excreted. If the blood becomes too highly concentrated, the kidney becomes overwhelmed and is unable to filter it. By measuring the sodium and osmolarity, the health care staff will know when the maximum amount of mannitol has been given. When this point is reached, other methods of lowering ICP must be used.

Another reason for measuring sodium and osmolarity levels is to look for signs of *specific* brain injuries. Head injury commonly causes disruption of the body's ability to regulate salt metabolism. There are three processes commonly seen in patients with head injury: cerebral salt wasting, diabetes insipidus, and SIADH. Cerebral salt wasting is a syndrome in which for unknown reasons the body is unable to retain sodium. The kidney expels the sodium out of the body when the patient urinates. This is not a problem with the kidney but rather a brain problem. The brain is unable to send the proper signals to the kidney so the kidney allows the salt to flow out of the body in the urine.

Diabetes insipidus is a problem with water regulation. In this process the brain sends improper signals to the kidney that results in water being wasted. When the kidney filters the blood, it allows a large amount of free water to pass out in the urine. Again, this is not a problem with the kidney but a problem in the brain. The kidney is just doing what the brain is telling it to do. The development of diabetes insipidus is an ominous sign in head injury. Patients who develop diabetes insipidus tend to be those with extremely severe brain injuries and these patients generally have a much poorer prognosis.

SIADH is the exact opposite of diabetes insipidus. In this process the brain sends a signal to the kidney to hold on to the water in the blood. The patient therefore produces a small amount of dark yellow urine with very little water in it. This condition can cause problems but is generally not as severe as diabetes insipidus. By restricting the amount of water the patient receives, the problem can easily be corrected.

What do the CT scan and MRI study tell you?

CT scans and MRI studies are incredibly valuable tools in patients with head injury. While a CT scan is generally more useful, there are times when MRI is needed. Both of these studies produce a detailed picture of the brain and ventricles. The CT scan is especially good at showing the bones of the face and skull. A CT scan is generally the test of choice in looking at the brain in trauma. It is performed more quickly than MRI and is very good at showing skull fractures and blood. The MRI study takes much longer to perform and therefore is not very useful in the acute period after the injury. Many of the patients are critically injured and cannot be left unattended for the amount of time necessary to complete an MRI study.

When a head injury patient arrives at the hospital, one of the first things done is a CT scan of the head. The CT scan provides the health care team with an excellent view of what is presently happening inside the patient's head. Skull fracture, brain **contusions,** and **subdural, epidural,** and **subarachnoid hemorrhages** are all easily detected with a CT scan. The CT scan can also show swelling, **edema,** and evidence of **herniation.** Once the CT scan is obtained, immediate decisions can be made as to which treatment is most appropriate. If the CT scan shows a large intracranial hemorrhage or open fracture, the patient will most likely be taken directly to the operating room. If the CT scan shows diffuse swelling or evidence of herniation, the patient is given mannitol immediately and taken to the ICU. CT scans are often repeated and it is not uncommon for a head injury patient to have many CT scans during the first few days of hospitalization.

MRI studies are rarely used in the immediate trauma setting. They simply take too long to obtain, and these critically ill patients cannot be left in the scanner for the 20 minutes it takes to complete the study. Another drawback is that MRI is not very good at showing bony injuries. The CT scan is quick and provides the health care team with all the information needed in the acute period.

Despite the limitations, MRI does have its place in caring for patients with head injury; it is unmatched at producing high-quality images of brain anatomy. MRI enables the physician to view the cerebral cortex, **cerebellum,** and **brain stem** in exquisite detail. Sometimes patients do not respond to therapy as expected. Further evaluation is required to determine exactly why these patients are not progressing. MRI can be used in these cases to look at the deep structures of the brain much more accurately than a CT scan. Specifically, injuries to the brain stem may not show up on a CT scan but are seen clearly with MRI. Not much can be done to correct brain stem injuries so finding them is not a priority in the acute setting (i.e., during the first 7 to 14 days after the injury). For this reason, CT is better in determining what needs to be done for the patient upon his or her arrival at the hospital.

MRI is most useful in the setting where patients have had a CT scan that does not seem to explain their clinical appearance. MRI may then reveal specific injuries in the brain stem that may not be correctable but may provide the health care team with valuable information regarding the likely course and outcome of the injury. In general, injuries to the brain stem are a serious problem and usually indicate significant long-term disability. Thus MRI provides prognostic information but usually does *not* give information that would change treatment.

Will the CT scan show how much brain damage there is?

The pictures produced by a CT scan are very good at showing the effects of damage on the brain. Usually a CT scan is all that is needed to evaluate the extent of intracranial damage from trauma. The CT images are limited though in terms of the relatively poor visualization of the cerebellum and brain stem. The pictures are detailed enough to tell the health care staff if surgery is indicated but quantifying the exact extent of injury is better done by MRI.

Will the CT scan tell you if the patient will wake up?

The images provided by CT and MRI may show damage in areas of the brain that control awareness but the predictive value of these pictures is unclear. Sometimes patients show significant damage to vital parts of their brain yet wake up and recover. The prognosis of any patient cannot be determined solely on the basis of a CT scan or MRI. The most important and sensitive measuring device of any neurologically injured patient is the neurologic examination performed by a physician. By combining the information gleaned by the neurologic examination with the CT and MRI pictures, the physician is often able to provide an idea about a patient's chance for improvement. Even this is not absolute and only the test of time will provide the answer to this question.

Why do some patients have multiple CT scans?

The introduction of the CT scan revolutionized the management of patients with head injury. In the past, physicians relied on the physical examination, plain x-ray films, and angiograms to create a picture of what was going on inside the patient's head. These tests are still important and the physical examination of the patient is still the most accurate tool for assessing the patient. The CT scan, however, provides a superior level of speed, accuracy, and detail that the other tests do not have. In about 30 seconds the physician is literally able to look inside the patient's head. By combining the CT picture with the physical examination the physician will be able to accurately diagnose the head injury patient in a matter of minutes. A process that used to take several minutes to hours can be completed in just a few minutes. The purpose of multiple CT scans is to follow the progression of intracranial injuries and identify any new ones. Often patients have small contusions or hematomas that are too small to warrant surgery. These patients will be followed with serial CT scans and regular neurologic assessments. By taking a number of pictures over time, the evolution or resolution of injuries can be followed. This allows the physician to intervene with therapy before the patient develops neurologic problems.

Another reason for repeating CT scans is that hydrocephalus, swelling, and strokes typically develop over a period of hours to days following an injury. A person may show clinical signs of a stroke but have a normal CT scan. If the CT scan is repeated the next day, the stroke may be seen in the area of brain that correlates with the neurologic deficit. Not every patient needs serial CT scans. Patients who show evidence of continued improvement generally do not need extra pictures of their healing brain. CT scans are very helpful but their use is dictated by the overall clinical picture of the patient.

Are there any risks in doing a CT scan?

CT scans are noninvasive tests. Basically, the CT scan machine uses x-rays to generate a detailed image of the brain. The risk of a CT scan comes from the radiation exposure. The radiation from a single CT scan is insignificant in terms of any long-term risk of developing radiation-induced cancer. The benefits of the CT scan in evaluating head injury patients far outweighs the relatively small, long-term risk due to exposure to the x-rays. The risks of the x-ray exposure from CT scans is more a factor in patients who are pregnant. Due to the risk of fetal abnormalities as a result of exposure to the x-rays, the abdomen is covered with a lead apron if a CT scan is absolutely necessary.

Another potential risk from CT scans has to do with the use of intravenous contrast material. This contrast material is a special dye injected into the veins that makes abnormal structures in the brain light up on the CT picture. This material can help sort out the different types of lesions known to affect the brain. For example, a brain tumor lights up in one way, whereas a stroke or hemorrhage has a much different pattern. The risk from this dye is that of an allergic reaction. Some people are very sensitive to the dye and can have kidney damage, seizures, or even cardiopulmonary arrest. Fortunately, intravenous dye is not frequently used in the management of head injury because traumatic brain damage tends to show up clearly without the use of dye.

Are there any risks in doing an angiogram?

There are two main risks associated with cerebral angiograms. The first is an allergic reaction to the dye that is injected. These allergic reactions can be minor, such as a rash, or much more severe. These allergic reactions are rare and the newer contrast materials have a lower risk than the dyes used in the past. People with allergies to seafood, particularly shellfish, tend to have a higher risk than people without these allergies.

The second risk to cerebral angiography is stroke. There is about a 1% chance of the patient having a stroke from the procedure. The manipulation of the catheter and injection of dye into the blood vessels can potentially cause small particles to break free of the internal wall (lumen) of a blood vessel and cause a stroke. The risk is low and angiograms are generally done only when the information they provide far exceeds the small risk of stroke.

Will the patient need a CT scan after being released from the hospital?

There is no simple answer to this question. Each patient's brain injury and therapy are unique. Some patients with head injuries will have a single CT scan and never need another one, while patients with more serious injuries may require multiple CT scans. Generally patients who have more than two CT scans while in the hospital eventually require another one sometime down the road. If the patient develops new or worsening neurologic symptoms after being released from the hospital, a CT scan is often obtained to make sure that there is nothing in the brain that requires treatment.

CHAPTER
5

Typical Symptoms
and Behavior

The various responses a patient displays to different clinical examinations are called neurologic signs. The combination of these signs indicates the overall health of the patient's brain, which is also called the patient's neurologic status. There is a wide range of neurologic signs that can occur with a head injury, each of which is used by the health care staff to estimate both the degree and location of the injury. Further, these signs can change from moment to moment as the injury process within the brain evolves. Therefore, it is important to examine the patient many times throughout the day, especially when the head injury is severe. By identifying any changes in the neurologic signs, the health care staff is able to ascertain the status of the patient at any given time and detect any deteriorations that may occur. A decline in the neurologic status of the patient may suggest that there is increased brain swelling or an expanding blood clot that needs to be removed surgically. Conversely, an improvement in the neurologic status usually suggests that the patient is beginning to recover.

AGITATION AND DISORDERS IN CONSCIOUSNESS

Agitation is very common in patients with head injury. In some instances the degree of agitation can be so excessive that it becomes dangerous for the patient. In these situations it may be necessary to give the patient medications that produce sedation, or even chemical **paralytics** for protection. This is particularly true for patients who also have a neck injury or those with significant **cerebral edema** (brain swelling). The extreme restlessness that occurs with severe agitation can worsen an unstable neck injury or increase **intracranial pressures** or **ICPs,** both of which are dangerous for the patient. The agitation most likely stems from the altered state of consciousness and confusion present in many head injury patients. Imagine waking up dazed from a deep sleep only to find yourself in a strange place (the **intensive care unit** or **ICU**) with monitors and tubes stuck into you. It is no wonder these patients are often agitated!

Head injury patients usually sustain a period of unconsciousness (the patient appears to be asleep) at the time of injury. This can vary in length from a few minutes to months or even years, depending on the severity of the head injury. In general, the longer the period of unconsciousness, the more severe the head injury. Although the patient may be unconscious, it does not necessarily mean that the brain and brain stem are completely inactive. The patient may still move around, either spontaneously or in response to a stimulus, despite being unconscious. That is to say that there are different categories, or layers, of unconsciousness. The unconscious state can be very deep or light enough so that the patient is only intermittently unconscious. The deepest and worst type of unconsciousness is when the patient shows *no activity at all* despite any stimuli, including deep pain. Such a result, in which there is no response at all, in the absence of any drugs that cause paralysis (inability to move) or recent seizure activity, is an extremely bad sign and suggests a very severe injury, especially if this condition persists. Most patients with an absence of any activity typically do not recover from the head injury to any appreciable degree.

DISORDERS IN MOVEMENT

While some patients may have no **motor activity,** or movements, when observed in a setting without any stimuli, they may move when a painful stimulus is applied. A significant stimulus is often necessary to elicit a response. In some cases the patient may exhibit a stereotypical response called **posturing.** Posturing is an automatic or reflexive movement in response to a stimulus. In general there are two types of posturing, **extending** and **flexing.** Both types of movement indicate damage in the connection between the brain and the brain stem. This unveils the more automatic movements controlled by the brain stem as the injured brain is no longer able to keep them under control. Extending occurs when the patient's

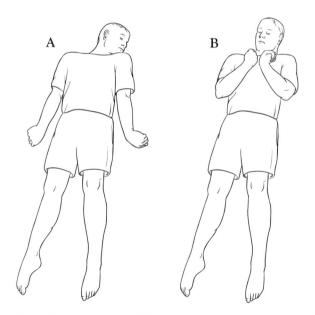

Figure 5-1 Examples of posturing. These responses occur when the brain is no longer able to control the brain stem. **A,** Extending, in which the patient's arms and legs are stiffly extended. The head also usually turns to one side. **B,** Flexing, in which the legs are also stiffly extended, but the arms are bent (i.e., flexed) at the elbow. Flexing is thought to represent a better response than extending in terms of expected outcomes.

arms and legs become very stiff and straighten out in response to a stimulus (Figure 5-1, A). This usually indicates that there is more damage to the brain stem than in patients who are flexing. Flexing is a condition in which the patient's legs are stiff and straightened out, similar to that which occurs in extending, but the arms bend at the elbow when a stimulus is applied (Figure 5-1, B).

Patients who are in a lighter state of unconsciousness may localize to a painful stimulus. This response, in which the patient moves a hand or arm to the location of the pain being applied, is called **localizing.** Such a response indicates a healthier brain and brain stem as opposed to that seen in posturing patients. This represents an important difference, since patients who localize tend to do better than those who exhibit posturing responses. Purposeful responses, in which the patient shows clear intent with individual movements, indicates a much lighter phase of unconsciousness (closer to being conscious rather than unconscious). Patients who are purposeful have an even better likelihood for a good recovery. Examples of purposeful movements include pulling the bed sheet up over the legs or body or attempting to pull out various tubes placed by the health care staff.

> **Ellen:** *Of course, my first question was, "Will my son be okay?" But you know, they can't tell that early, it can go either way. He had a lot of swelling, but he was responding to finger commands and so on. A male nurse came in and said, "Steve gave me the finger." And I said, "Oh, my God, I am sorry, I am so sorry." He laughed, "Oh no, this is great progress! He's showing us that he's aggravated that we keep telling him to move this and move that."*

The movements described above are usually symmetric in that they occur equally on both sides of the body. This may not be the case if there is damage to the areas of the brain that control movement. Injury to specific portions of the frontal cortex can result in weakness in the face, arm, or leg on the opposite side of the body. This is due to the cross wiring in the nervous system such that one

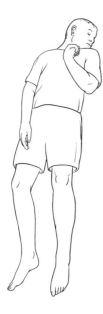

Figure 5-2 Hemiplegia superimposed on posturing. Some injuries can result in the inability to move one side while also producing posturing responses. In this illustration, the patient displays flexing on the left side of the body while the right side remains limp.

side of the brain controls the opposite side of the body. Extensive injury to the frontal lobe can result in the inability to move the entire opposite side of the body, termed **hemiplegia.** This type of injury can be superimposed on other clinical signs of brain or brain stem damage. For example, a patient with hemiplegia who is posturing will only show the stereotypical movement on one side of the body, while the other side does not move at all (Figure 5-2). Hemiplegia can also occur with injuries to the brain stem that damage the motor connections between the brain and the body.

DISORDERS FROM BRAIN STEM INJURY

The brain stem is a vitally important structure, due to the multiple reciprocal connections between the brain and body that run through it. There are also multiple control centers located within the brain stem, including the life control center located in the medulla, and the **ascending reticular activating system** or **ARAS,** which is involved in maintaining consciousness. The brain stem, however, is relatively small in size despite all that it contains. Hence, small areas of damage can produce large functional deficits since the multiple connections in the brain stem are all very close to each other. Any number of deficits may result from damage to the brain stem.

Injury to the uppermost portion of the brain stem, called the **midbrain,** can damage the ARAS, resulting in unconsciousness. The ARAS, which is a combination of many centers in the brain, helps to initiate and maintain consciousness. Very simplistically speaking, it is the system that wakes up the brain. The center that controls the size of the pupils may also be affected; the affected pupil will be large and dilated (Figure 5-3). Another center located nearby controls different eye movements. Patients who have damage to this center may not be able to move the eyes in certain directions. Damage lower down in the brain stem, in the **pons,** can result in the inability to feel one side of the face. The face may also appear to droop if the facial movement center is damaged. This sensory deficit can also affect the clear covering of the eye called the cornea. The normal protective blink reflex, called the **corneal reflex,** may be lost in these situations.

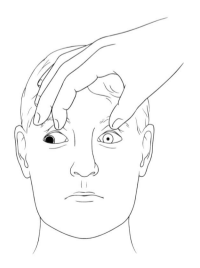

Figure 5-3   A "blown" right pupil. The right pupil is dilated and does not get smaller in bright light. This can occur with injury to the midbrain or oculomotor nerve (third nerve), or from direct damage to the eye itself. When a patient develops a "new" blown pupil (i.e., one that was not present initially after the accident), it may be a sign of impending herniation.

There is also a control center located within the pons that helps move the eyes together in tandem. Injury to this area may result in the inability to move eyes together called **dysconjugate gaze.** Injuries to the **medulla** can damage the life control center, which can be devastating, as the ability to breathe automatically may be permanently lost. Loss of blood pressure control and heart beat can be equally devastating to the patient because damage to this portion of the brain stem usually results in death. Less extensive injury to the medulla can result in the loss of the protective **gag reflex.**

SPEECH DISORDERS

As discussed in Chapter 2, the function of speech is spread out in different portions of the dominant side (the left side in the majority of patients) of the brain. Different abnormalities of language may occur, depending on which part of the "speech" brain is injured. Damage to the frontal lobe can result in the inability to make word sounds, such that when the patient attempts to speak, the sounds produced are garbled, as if the patient has a mouth full of marbles. While the patient may be able to make the word sounds correctly, the actual content (making sentences out of words) may be mixed up and disordered. This occurs with damage to the dominant parietal lobe, which can also cause the inability to understand speech. Such speech abnormalities are collectively called **aphasias.**

VISUAL ABNORMALITIES

Because the visual system is spread throughout the brain, it is uncommon to completely lose vision from the traumatic damage that occurs in head injury. The exception is if there is significant damage to both **occipital lobes** or both eyes. Extensive injury in these areas can result in total loss of vision. Although this can happen, it is uncommon to have irreversible damage to both eyes or both occipital lobes from head injury. More commonly injuries result in the inability to see part of the visual field (Figure 5-4). For example,

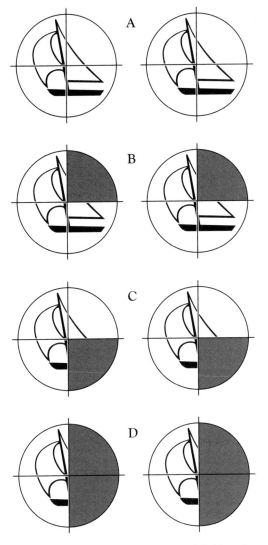

Figure 5-4   Visual field abnormalities. The "visual field" refers to what is seen with each eye. The images collected by each eye are then superimposed by the occipital lobes to produce a three-dimensional view. In this illustration, a sailboat is being visualized. **A,** Normal visual fields. **B,** Superior quadranopsia, where the upper outer portion of the visual field is not visualized, as may occur with damage to the temporal lobes. **C,** Inferior quadranopsia, which can occur with damage to the parietal lobes. **D,** Hemianopsia, where one entire side of the visual field is lost.

damage to one of the occipital lobes can lead to the inability to see half of the visual field. This is called **hemianopsia.** Injury to the temporal lobe, which affects the connections from the eyes to the occipital lobe, may result in a less extensive loss of the visual field. Such injuries typically result in **superior quadranopsia,** in which the patient cannot see the upper outer portion of the visual field. Similarly, damage to the parietal lobe can result in the inability to see the lower outer portion of the visual field, termed **inferior quad-ranopsia.** While such deficits can initially be bothersome, patients often learn to compensate quite well for these partial visual losses.

While not actually a visual loss, injury to the frontal lobe can result in the inability to look to one side. Patients with this type of injury cannot make the eyes move to the opposite side. The eyes appear locked or stuck on one side. This is similar to what occurs when there is damage to the "lateral gaze center" in the pons (Figure 5-5).

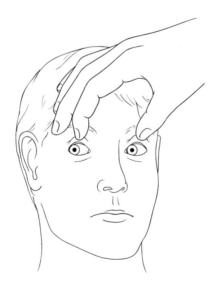

Figure 5-5 Lateral gaze abnormality. The eyes are "stuck" looking to the right. This can occur with damage to the right frontal lobe or to the brain stem.

Donna: *Sharon still has double vision from the injury and we thought she was going to need surgery. Fortunately, she was prescribed special glasses with prisms so she can see without shutting one eye or wearing a patch.*

ASSOCIATED INJURIES

Significant forces are typically involved in head injuries, particularly those as a result of a motor vehicle accident. One look at a vehicle involved in a serious collision is all it takes to understand just how much force can be involved. Although the car often absorbs much of the impact, the passengers inside are also subjected to a certain degree of the impact, depending on the type and circumstances of the accident. This leads to broken bones in the arms, legs, face, and pelvis; injury to internal organs, such as the heart, lungs, liver, kidneys, and spleen; and bruising and swelling **(edema)** of the soft tissue in the entire body, including the head and face. It is this bruising and swelling, especially in the head and face, that can impart a ghastly appearance to head injury patients. It is important to remember, however, that both the bruising and swelling are temporary and will resolve with time. In addition, although the head and face may be terribly swollen, this does not necessarily reflect the status of the brain. The brain may be fine despite massive swelling of the eyes, face, and head.

Another striking, potential feature seen in head injury patients are convulsions or seizures. A seizure is the result of excessive and disorganized electrical activity inside the brain. Areas of brain damage can short-circuit the normal electrical activity leading to the development of seizures. Different kinds of convulsions can occur in head injury patients. These range from shaking of the entire body (a **grand mal seizure**) to uncontrollable shaking in just one part of the body. Some attacks occur in which there is no body movement at all. Sometimes one type can spread within the brain and become another type, often ending up in grand mal activity. Patients who have an attack are usually very still and unconscious for a period of time after the seizure ceases. It is important, although not always possible, to prevent these since they can cause more damage in the already-damaged brain.

THE PERSONNEL

To handle the variety of injuries that may be present in these patients, multiple surgical teams, from different specialties, typically become involved in the care of the patient. This provides specialized attention and treatment for each particular injury. Family members, however, can easily become confused as they meet or hear the names of the many physicians involved in the case. Family members may have occasion to speak with **neurosurgeons** (brain and spine specialists), **orthopedists** (bone specialists), **trauma surgeons** (surgeons involved with the treatment of the internal organ injury), and **anesthesiologists** (the specialists who put patients to "sleep" for surgical procedures). In order to keep track of all these surgical teams, the family members should ask, "What type of doctor are you?" By identifying the different specialties involved, it may help to understand the extent of the patient's injuries and decrease the confusion from seeing so many physicians.

The number of people involved in the total care of the patient extends beyond the physicians and nurses. Many head injury patients will also be seen by physical and occupational therapists who attempt to help the patient regain function with extensive therapy. Nutritionists often become involved as well, making sure that the patient is meeting all the necessary food and dietary requirements to aid in the recovery process. Respiratory therapists ensure that the ventilator is working correctly and may administer inhaled medications. Again, if family members become confused by the sheer number of people coming and going from the room, they should ask them to explain what they are doing. Most health care staff personnel are more than willing to stop and talk with family members.

⸙ COMMONLY ASKED QUESTIONS ⸙

What are the warning signs of a significant head injury?

Almost everyone at one time or another has witnessed or been the victim of a minor head injury. These injuries can range from a simple bump on the head to something more serious in which consciousness is affected. People with minor head trauma often do not even see a physician and are just fine. Not every bump on the head requires medical attention. The things to look for in a person with a seemingly minor head injury that should prompt a visit to the emergency departments are as follows:

- Person is overly sleepy and difficult to wake up
- Blurry vision or severe headache
- Repeat episodes of vomiting and/or nausea
- Clear fluid dripping from ears or nose
- Difficulty with walking or balance
- Poor or incoherent speech, memory, and/or confusion
- Weakness or sensory changes in the arms, face, or legs.
- Abnormal body movements

These are general guidelines to look out for in a person who has been hit in the head. If any of the above signs or symptoms develop, the person should be taken to the nearest emergency department as soon as possible. Another guideline is if the person "just doesn't look right." Many times we are unable to describe or recognize exactly what is wrong with someone but get a feeling that something is wrong. If this happens to be the case, the person should be brought to the emergency department. Remember, the brain is very delicate and does not tolerate injury well. Always err on the side of caution and if any doubt exists, bring the person to medical attention.

Have the patient's eyes opened?

Patients who have severe head injury typically have prolonged periods of unconsciousness, during which time the eyes are usually closed. Patients with less severe head injury or those recovering from severe head injury may have periods where they appear to be more awake followed by periods of being more lethargic. This can be viewed as a sign that, although the brain is not entirely healthy, it is beginning to recover, especially if the periods of alertness lengthen. During those periods of being more "awake" the eyes may open.

Some patients may not open their eyes unless they are given some stimulus (often a painful one), while others simply cannot open their eyes due to major swelling around the eyes. Conversely, patients who are deeply unconscious may appear to have their eyes open due to swelling of the eyeballs, which forces the eyelids open. These patients typically appear to be blankly staring off into space. The key is that eye opening and the level of consciousness do not always go hand-in-hand. A patient can be almost fully awake but not open the eyes, while another who is completely unconscious may have the eyes open.

Can the patient hear us?

This is an interesting question, since what actually gets through to the patient on some level during unconsciousness is unknown. The problem is that consciousness and unconsciousness most likely have different levels, although this is not truly known. There have been accounts of patients recalling something that was said to them or some continual "beeping noise" from one of the various monitors while they were unconscious. This remains one of the many unknowns in patients with head injury, and most likely varies from patient to patient. Given this, it certainly cannot hurt to talk to the patient on the chance that something is getting through on some level.

More specifically, it must be remembered that the ears and the nerves that carry the sounds to the brain must be working. Skull fractures can cut the hearing nerve in half or damage it to a degree that the patient cannot hear out of the affected ear. Although very uncommon, both hearing nerves could be damaged in such a way as to leave the patient unable to hear. Other factors, such as blood within the ear, can also temporarily decrease the ability to hear, but this disability resolves itself when the blood is no longer present.

Does the patient know we are here?

Given the uncertainties of what is actually going on in a patient's brain during unconsciousness, this is difficult to answer for certain. If the patient appears to show signs of increased activity in your presence, this may be a subtle indication that you are recognized in some way. Such signs of increased activity might range from an obvious increase in the movements of the body, to something subtle, such as an unexplained increase in the heart rate, breathing rate, or blood pressure (these changes can be seen on the telemetry monitor above the patient) due to your presence; it is difficult to tell for certain.

> **Sarah:** *I spent a lot of time talking to Jim about the kids and the farm while he was in a coma. Often it would make his rates go up because he would get so excited. Sometimes they didn't want me in there very long! I think my visits were limited to about 10 minutes in the ICU.*

Can the patient breathe?

Most patients with head injury are able to breathe on their own. Many, however, are too confused to protect their airway and need to use a ventilator. Some patients have other injuries to their lungs that require time to heal. The breathing machine is a way to support the lungs until patients are able to once again do their job.

Some of the most severe brain injuries involve the parts of the brain that tell our lungs to take a breath. The automatic breathing response is broken so the lungs don't get the signal from the brain telling them to breathe. These patients would suffocate without the breathing machine. This type of injury is extremely serious and many of these patients do not survive.

Is the patient in pain?

There is little question about this in patients who are more or less awake since they can answer the question themselves. In patients who are less responsive, it is more difficult to tell. In certain instances the presence of pain can be inferred by an increase in the heart rate or blood pressure when the effects of a previously administered pain medication wear off. There are many medications that can be given to relieve even the worst pain when it is thought that the patient is uncomfortable. Those who are deeply unconscious are most likely not in any pain. Although they may have multiple injuries, such as broken bones and ribs, internal organ damage, and bruises all over the body; injuries that would certainly be very painful to a patient who is fully awake, the sensation or awareness of pain requires a certain degree of consciousness.

It should be noted that there are no pain receptors in the brain tissue. In other words, a cut or bruise in the brain does not cause pain to the patient (although such a maneuver could cause some loss of function). The pain that a patient feels is from the injuries throughout the body, not from the bruises, swelling, or damage that are in the brain itself.

Why does the patient become agitated?

Imagine waking up from a deep sleep to find yourself in a strange place with tubes, catheters, and wires connected to you. Now imagine that when you awaken you are not fully alert but still somewhat groggy. The confusion of the new setting, combined with not being fully awake, can lead to a degree of agitation. This, in a sense, is the situation with head injury patients. They find themselves in the ICU with no idea how they got there, wires and tubes protruding from their bodies, and, at the least, a pretty bad headache. Those with small children can attest that sometimes upon awakening a child from a deep sleep, the child shows much the same signs of agitation. The situation with head injury patients is similar, only multiplied many times over. Further, in some patients, the injury damages the portions of the brain that give us our adult or mature qualities. Depending on the degree and location of injury, damage can result in primitive or child-like behavior and significant agitation. While it can be difficult for families to see the patient in an agitated state, it is a relatively good sign that the brain is not horribly damaged. It is certainly better to see a patient agitated and actively moving around, exhibiting purposeful movements, than it is to see a patient quiet and motionless. The agitation and spontaneous movements are signs that the brain is reacting and, although not necessarily appropriate, they are signs that the brain is functioning on some level. Patients who are quiet and motionless are much more at risk, since this may suggest that the brain is not functioning very well.

What is brain herniation? What causes it?

According to the American Heritage Dictionary the word herniate means "protrusion of a bodily structure through the wall that normally contains it." Brain herniation refers to an event in which a portion of the brain is pushed or swells out of its normal location, usually subsequent to being pressed up against the brain stem. Herniation can be caused by any head injury that causes increased ICP. The injury may be diffuse, as in the shearing-type of head injury, or localized such as with an **epidural hematoma.** Any injury that creates a situation that leads to displacement of normal brain structures can lead to herniation.

The problem is that the brain is very soft and thus can be moved around within the skull. As damaged areas, such as contusions or expanding blood clots, begin to enlarge, the brain may be pushed out of its normal position. Similarly, in situations where the entire brain is swollen or the ICP is very high, the outer portions of the brain, which are pushed up against the skull, begin to compress the inner parts of the brain. As the brain begins to shift within the skull cavity, areas not initially injured can become compressed. This compression can lead to damage of these normal portions of the brain. Once the compression of the brain, either by an expanding damaged area or secondary to elevated ICPs, is significant enough, the brain stem begins to become compressed. As the abnormally swollen brain begins surrounding the brain stem it begins to strangle it. The blood supply to the brain stem becomes compromised, which can lead to irreversible damage to the brain stem. If the life control centers within the brain stem cease to function, the patient will die.

Is herniation reversible? Can you test for it?

Herniation refers to a sequence of events that occurs over a period of a few seconds to minutes. The reversibility of herniation is dependent on early recognition, rapid intervention, and the existence of a reversible cause. All patients at risk of herniation are placed in an ICU where they are constantly monitored by nurses and doctors specially trained to recognize the early warning signs of herniation. If a patient shows signs of herniation, the next step is to take immediate steps to reverse it. This may include any or all of the following treatments. The patient is given a large dose of mannitol, have a ventriculostomy placed, be hyperventilated, or may even be taken for emergency surgical decompression. The reversibility is often dependent on the underlying cause of the herniation. Sometimes the damage is too extensive or progresses too rapidly to enable life-saving intervention. In some instances herniation can be halted if it is recognized and treated rapidly.

The best method to predict and rapidly identify signs of herniation is by regularly following the patient's neurologic examination. A relatively quick decline in the patient's neurologic examination, with the patient subsequently exhibiting extensor posturing and developing a nonreactive pupil to light, is a warning sign that herniation is beginning to occur. Other helpful monitoring devices are Camino monitors, ventriculostomies, and CT scans. The information obtained by all of these modalities can help the health care team closely follow the progression of the intracranial process. Following the trend in each of these measurements will hopefully make it possible to intervene before herniation begins.

Does herniation mean that the patient will die?

Herniation describes a process in which the brain is being displaced and compressing vital structures (usually the brain stem). If the process cannot be reversed, for whatever reason, the patient will go on to completely herniate. The patient who is said to have "herniated" typically does not recover. The displacement of the brain in these instances is typically so severe that the vital centers of the brain stem that control breathing and consciousness have been wiped out. Such patients will not recover from the herniation. A simple comparison is with the verb "to drown." A person who is drowning can be saved. A person who has drowned cannot be saved.

Why are the patient's movements jerky? Are these permanent?

There are a variety of different movements a patient can make that might be described as jerky movements. Some of the movements are expected and easily explained, while others may indicate something more ominous. Head injury patients who are conscious are often seen having jerky movements when trying to perform a specific task. These uncoordinated movements may be a result of damage to the cerebellum or cortical motor areas, parts of the brain that help to control movement. These patients need to relearn how to do things because the circuitry of the brain has changed because of the injury. With aggressive physical therapy patients often overcome their disability and their movements typically become more fluid.

Another type of jerky movement seen in head injury patients is the tonic shaking of seizures. These movements are often scary for family members because the patient may violently shake with strange eye movements and sounds. Seizures tend to last anywhere from seconds to minutes and are caused by cortical (i.e., brain injuries) or metabolic (i.e., chemical or electrolyte) abnormalities. It is important to attempt to control such seizures with medication because persistent seizures can be very damaging to the healing brain. Many head injury patients are placed on anticonvulsant medication to prevent seizures.

Sometimes seizures may be subtle and are manifested by a rhythmic beating of the hand. In these instances it may not be clear whether the patient is actually having a seizure. In these cases an EEG may be helpful in determining whether the patient is having seizure activity.

Another form of shaking is termed "myoclonus," a situation in which the patient experiences sudden, uncontrollable muscle contractions. The contractions tend to be random but most commonly affect the muscles of the limbs. They are very common in patients who have suffered a period of hypoxia. There is no specific treatment for these movements, in contrast to seizures, but their frequency tends to subside as the patient recovers.

What causes paralysis?

Paralysis describes the inability to move. This can affect one or more limbs, as well as the face and eyes. Damage to different areas within the brain, brain stem, and spinal cord can all produce various types of paralysis. The common denominator for these paralytic injuries is that each involves some type of injury to the motor system (i.e., the system responsible for moving the various parts of the body). This system consists of portions of the **frontal lobe** within the brain, the brain stem, and the spinal cord. The frontal lobe is the location where the commands to move originate. This center sends impulses through the brain stem into the spinal cord, telling it which muscles to move. The spinal cord then sends impulses to the muscles, making them move.

In other words, the brain produces the blueprint to move and the spinal cord carries out the job. The brain stem carries the information from the brain to the spinal cord. Damage at any point in this motor system can interrupt this pathway and result in paralysis.

Injury to the one frontal lobe can produce hemiplegia (the inability to move one side of the body). The paralysis in this case affects the opposite side of the body. The same can occur with injury to the spinal cord or brain stem. Damage to both sides of the brain stem or spinal cord can produce complete paralysis (i.e., inability to move either side of the body) called paraplegia. The higher the damage in the spinal cord, the more portions of the body that are paralyzed. For example, injuries to the spinal cord in the mid to lower back may result in the inability to move the legs and bladder, while an injury to the spinal cord in the neck may result in the inability to move the arms or legs. In these injuries the brain is working fine but it cannot get the messages to move through to the body.

Why is the patient so swollen?

Critically ill patients often are sustained by the use of intravenous fluids, blood transfusions, and tube feedings. Many of these patients also have multiple metabolic problems that create an abnormal nutritional environment. The fluids within the body are primarily blood and water. The blood is made up of red and white blood cells, proteins, salt, and minerals. During a serious traumatic injury the normal balance of water in the bloodstream is altered. Many times in order to keep the blood pressure stable, intravenous fluids and blood must be given to the patient at a fast rate. Once the patient is stabilized, the rate of infusion of these fluids can be slowed. During an extended time in the ICU, many patients appear puffy or swollen. The puffiness results from water leaving the bloodstream and collecting in the muscle, skin, and fat. The swelling usually goes away once the patient's need for fluids has passed.

What types of changes can be expected from the frontal lobe injury?

The frontal lobes are involved in many different functions, including bodily movements, eye movements from side to side, and speech production. The frontal lobes are also thought to be involved with personality, motivation, social appropriateness, and higher thought functions. Because of the multiple functions that the frontal lobes help to control, damage to these lobes produces a somewhat unpredictable constellation of deficits. Further, different patients appear to respond differently to damage in the frontal lobes. Some patients show definite alterations in various aspects of their behavior, while others with the identical amount of damage show little to no alterations or deficits.

Given this climate of uncertainty, some general information regarding frontal lobe injury follows. The center from where the commands to move the body originate is located toward the back of the frontal lobe, where the frontal lobe and parietal lobe meet. Damage to this location can lead to hemiplegia on the opposite side of the body. The severity of this deficit can vary, in that only the arm, leg, or face is affected, while the other limbs function normally. Damage located on the side of the dominant frontal lobe can produce the inability to produce speech (i.e., aphasia). These patients can understand speech as well as read and write, but they cannot get their vocal apparatus to produce the necessary sounds to generate speech. In other words, they appear to be tongue-tied, which can be very frustrating, as they know what they want to say but they just can't quite say it. Damage to either side of the frontal lobes can also produce lateral eye movement abnormalities. This area of the frontal lobes controls movement of both the eyes from side to side. This system is crossed so that the right frontal lobe makes the eyes look to the left and vice versa for the left frontal lobe. Significant damage to one side of a frontal lobe results in the inability to move the eyes to the opposite side. For example, damage to the right frontal lobe can result in the eyes appearing stuck looking to the right side. This is because the damaged area cannot get the eyes to look over to the opposite side.

As indicated earlier, the frontal lobe is also thought to be involved with behavior, motivation, personality, and higher thought functions. These functions are generally thought to be located on the undersurface of the frontal lobes. Damage to this area, which is fairly common in severe head injuries, can produce a variety of behavior and personality alterations. Such information comes from previous individuals who have suffered damage to these areas. Some patients have shown an almost complete lack of any type of motivation, in which they do not eat, do not maintain any type of personal hygiene, and do not move or speak. This particular syndrome represents an example of what very extensive injury to the frontal lobes can produce. More often patients have less severe alterations in behavior where some may appear more docile while others appear disinhibited. Damage to the frontal lobes can also decrease the patient's ability to participate in complex thinking as well as performing more complicated tasks. The ability to concentrate is also commonly affected.

What are reflexes?

Reflexes are the body's automatic reactions to different stimuli. When a person accidentally places a hand on something very hot, the hand is quickly removed before it is badly burned. This is a reflex movement in that it occurs automatically without any thought. There are many different reflexes, some more complex than others, that help protect and enable us to function properly during everyday life. The brain and brain stem also have reflexes that can be tested to assess how well these structures are functioning. These are particularly important in patients who are unconscious since they cannot voluntarily cooperate with an examination. These reflexes include constriction of the pupils when a light is shown in the eye **(pupillary reflex),** the automatic movement of the eyes when the head is turned from side to side **(doll's eyes response),** and the gag response when the back of the throat is touched with a cotton swab, or when the breathing tube **(endotracheal tube)** is gently moved back and forth. There are other reflex movements that occur in patients who are unconscious. These include withdrawing the leg when the bottom of the foot is stroked with an object, pulling the arms and hands toward the face after a painful stimulus is applied, or moving the hands and arms toward the feet after application of a painful stimulus to the patient's body.

Using knowledge of anatomy, the presence or absence of these various reflexes can help determine which portions of the brain stem are functioning properly. Damage to the brain stem, even small areas, can be devastating to the patient. Injury to the portion of the brain stem considered the life support center (the medulla) can be fatal. Therefore, the continued assessment of these various reflexes is used to determine what damage has already occurred and to watch for any change in the injury. The loss of certain reflexes, or the development of reflexes that were not originally present, suggests that something is changing, sometimes for the worse, sometimes for the better.

What is posturing?

In general, posturing is an abnormal movement that occurs secondary to damage to the brain and/or the brain stem. There are two broad types, flexing and extending, which are actually reflex movements normally suppressed by the brain. In other words, these reflex movements are not present in a patient with a normal brain and brain stem. Flexing, also called **decorticate posturing,** describes a response in which the patient bends the arms at the elbows and stiffly straightens the legs in response to a painful stimulus. When the patient stiffly straightens the arms and legs, it is termed extending or **decerebrate posturing.** The centers responsible for these reflex movements are located in the brain stem. When the brain is no longer able to keep these centers under control, either from injury to the brain itself or from an injury to the brain stem that no longer allows the brain to communicate with these centers in the brain stem, these two reflex centers in the brain stem are unleashed. Depending on the location of the injury, either flexing or extending posturing may be exhibited by the patient in response to stimuli.

The presence of posturing responses to stimuli indicates that there is severe injury in the brain and/or the brain stem and this, therefore, is not a good sign. Flexing is better than extending as it suggests that the injury is farther away from the life control center in the brain stem. Patients who change from exhibiting flexing posturing to extending are thought to be getting worse. The implication is that the damage in the brain stem is extending down through the brain stem toward the life control center, a center that, if damaged, results in the patient's death.

Why are the patient's pupils unequal?

Normally the pupils become smaller when a bright light is shone into the eyes. You can see this if you stand in front of a mirror, turn off the lights, then turn them back on. The pupils quickly get smaller. This is an automatic response to bright light called the pupillary reflex. This reflex is controlled by the upper most portion of the brain stem called the midbrain. The nerves sent from the midbrain, called the **third nerves (oculomotor nerves),** to the eyes help to control the size of the pupils (the black portion located in the center of the eyes). There are other nerves that go to the eyes causing the pupils to get larger. These two nerves work together to control the size of the pupil. Damage to the oculomotor nerve (the constrictor nerve) prevents the pupil from getting smaller when bright light is shone in the affected eye. If the oculomotor nerve to one eye is working while the other one is not, the pupil in the eye with the injured nerve appears larger than the pupil in the normal eye (see Figure 5-3). This is because the nerve to the eye that increases the size of the pupil still works, even though the nerve that decreases the size of the pupil does not. The eye with the large pupil is called a "blown pupil." This is a very important finding used by the health care staff to evaluate the patient because this may be a sign that the pressure within the brain is dangerously high.

The development of an unequal or blown pupil (i.e., a pupil that does not get smaller with bright lights) in a patient who previously had normal pupils is considered a neurosurgical emergency. The development of a blown pupil may indicate that the nerves to the eye are being compressed, a sign of impending herniation. Herniation can quickly lead to compression of the life control center and death. This is why the nurses and physicians always seem to be shining a flashlight into a patient's eyes. They are making sure the pupils are reacting appropriately to the light.

Injury to the midbrain, the portion of the brain stem that helps control the pupil size via the oculomotor nerves, can also lead to a dilated or blown pupil. In this instance the damage to the pupil control center rather than the nerves causes the larger pupil. The difference is that the injury to the midbrain usually occurs at the time of the injury. Therefore, the affected pupil is large right after the accident as opposed to impending herniation, in which the pupil gets large (or "blown") a certain period of time *after* the accident. Little can be done for the injury that occurs to the midbrain at the time of the accident. Thus it is the timing of when the pupil gets large. If it is large right after the accident, it suggests midbrain injury, which will hopefully normalize with time. This can also happen when there is direct damage to the eye itself. Serious injury to the eye may result in the damage of the nerves right at the pupil, which may also cause a large or dilated pupil. Again, the pupil is usually large right after the accident. The development of a nonreactive pupil later, after the accident, suggests another problem, namely impending herniation, which is an emergency requiring immediate treatment.

What happens in temporal lobe injury?

Temporal lobe injuries are not uncommon in head injuries, particularly those secondary to motor vehicle accidents. The temporal lobe, located just behind and slightly below the frontal lobe, is one area within the brain that is particularly prone to developing seizure activity. Patients with damage to this lobe are definitely at risk for developing seizures. Seizure activity that results from temporal lobe injury can be short-lived in that the seizure activity stops after certain period of time after the accident, or it can persist for years after the accident. Most patients are given **anticonvulsants,** medications designed to prevent seizures, for the first week or so after the accident. Patients who continue to have seizures require the medication for a longer period of time.

The temporal lobes are also thought to be involved in the formation of new memories. Memory can be generally divided into long-term and short-term. The short-term memory functions, in which forming new memories is a feature, are thought to be in large part controlled by the temporal lobes. Damage to these lobes in some instances can decrease a patient's ability to form new memories. The memories stored prior to the damage usually remain intact. In other words, although the mechanism used to store new information is dysfunctional, the information already stored can still be retrieved. For example, a patient with temporal lobe damage may forget a new acquaintance's name but remember a family member's name without difficulty.

An important consideration in patients with temporal lobe injury is the fact that the temporal lobe is very close to the brain stem. The life control center, crucial in maintaining life, is located in the brain stem. Due to the proximity of the temporal lobe to the brain stem, any swelling in the temporal lobe can result in compression of the brain stem. This is why patients with relatively large areas of damage, such as contusions, in the temporal lobe are watched very closely. They are at risk for compression of the brain stem and subsequent herniation.

CHAPTER

6

⎯⎯⎯⎯⎯⎯•⎯⎯⎯⎯⎯⎯

Surgical Management: What It Can Do and How It's Done

Some, but not all, types of head injury require and respond to surgical intervention. The shearing injury described in Chapter 3 is one type of injury that generally does not respond to surgical intervention. It is a diffuse cellular injury, deep within the brain, that cannot be fixed by surgery. Other injuries, such as epidural, subdural, and some contusions, are readily treated surgically. The success of surgery is often dependent on the time between the initial injury and the surgical intervention.

In general, brain surgery is limited by the constraints placed on the surgeon by the anatomy of the brain. Some areas are vital for neurologic function and surgical removal of them may save the patient's life but leave him or her neurologically devastated, such that the life saved would be one of minimal to no function. Surgery can be very effective when there are discrete injuries in noneloquent (i.e., less vital) areas. Contusions and hematomas can often be removed with relatively little damage to the surrounding brain. The neurosurgeon is guided by the principle of "saving brain." The surgeon operates as soon as possible, saving the brain from further compressive damage caused by a hematoma. During the operation the surgeon is ever mindful of protecting the noninjured and vital areas of the brain. Most of the operations done for brain trauma are variations of a single operation. This operation, the craniotomy, is described, as are other surgical procedures commonly used to treat brain trauma patients.

> **Sarah:** At about 5:30 the morning after the accident, a scan showed that Jim had a clot and an abrasion, where part of the skull had actually punctured a part of the brain. . . . The surgeon came into the waiting room before surgery eager to go. . . . We were fortunate . . . Jim got into surgery first thing before all the previously scheduled surgeries were due to begin . . . this was all quite difficult to absorb.

Each traumatic brain injury is unique in that the exact location, size, and number of hemorrhages are never the same. The operation performed must be tailored to the injuries inside each particular patient's head. The operation in general is referred to as a "craniotomy," but each one is a little bit different because no two injuries are *exactly* the same. Craniotomy means opening the cranium (skull). The specific site on the skull where the opening is made is dependent on where the underlying damage is located. The operative techniques vary in different areas of the brain. Some areas can be taken out completely without any damage to the patient; more eloquent (i.e., critical) areas cannot even be approached by the surgeon without leaving the patient badly injured. Many examples of operative strategy and techniques will be described later as they relate to specific injuries. To begin, a general description of the common steps in virtually every craniotomy follows.

CRANIOTOMY

After shaving the head or a portion of the head, the scalp is disinfected with a standard surgical antiseptic solution. A marker is used to draw the planned incision on the scalp. A rather large incision is made in the shape of an arch or a question mark behind the patient's hairline (Figure 6-1). This creates a flap of skin that is folded over and held in place by special clamps. Once the skin has been peeled back, the skull and temporalis muscle can be seen (Figure 6-2). The temporalis muscle is located on the side of the head just in front of the ear. If you place your hand on the side of your head half way between your ear and eye and then bite down, you will feel the temporalis contract. This muscle is divided and folded over with the skin flap and held out of the way with clamps. Because the temporalis is a muscle used for chewing, after a craniotomy, some patients complain of pain when eating.

Once these steps have been accomplished, the skull is the next barrier faced by the surgeon. A drill is used to make two or three small holes ("burr holes") in the skull. The **dura** can be seen at the bottom of each hole. A flat dissecting tool is used to separate the dura from the edges of the burr hole. A special attachment is placed on the drill, which is then placed into the burr hole and used to cut a round flap out of the skull. The drill attachment is designed such that it travels between the undersurface of the skull and above the dura. This is to ensure that neither the dura nor the underlying brain is damaged by the drill. Once this is done, the bone flap is easily removed, much like taking a piece out of a puzzle (Figure 6-3). These are the beginning steps for most craniotomies.

Once the head is opened, the operation is individualized to meet the needs of the specific patient. There are some techniques common to all brain operations, but the surgical plan and decisions made are directly related to the patient's type of brain injury. For instance, operating on a subdural hematoma requires a different surgical approach than a gunshot wound. The brief description of the surgical techniques and principles for a variety of injuries that follow is not meant to be an account of the surgeries in detail, but rather a description of the surgeon's rationale for what is done in the operating room.

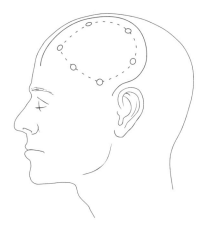

Figure 6-1 The general question mark shape of most incisions made in craniotomies performed for head injury. The location of the burr holes and their connections (i.e., the circles and dotted lines) for the bone flap are also shown.

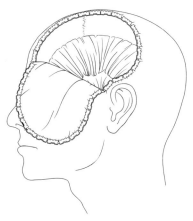

Figure 6-2 First step to a craniotomy. The skin flap exposes the underlying temporalis muscle ("chewing muscle") and skull. Small clips are placed on the skin margins to prevent bleeding.

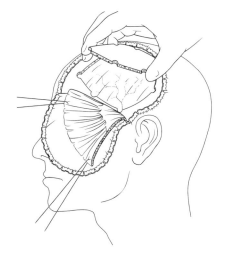

Figure 6-3 Removal of the bone flap. Once the skin and temporalis muscle have been moved out of the way, the skull is exposed. Burr holes are then made in the bone with a drill. These are connected, making a bone flap. The bone flap is removed, exposing the underlying dura.

Epidural Hematoma

This is one of the more straightforward operations done for trauma. **Epidural hematomas** often result from seemingly minimal trauma. They result from a small amount of force applied to a vulnerable area of the skull, typically just below the temporal bone on the side of the head. This region is often referred to by nonmedical people as the temple. The bone in this area is the temporal bone; it is very thin in some parts, and it can be very easily fractured. A large artery courses just below the bone and can be injured or cut by the sharp edge of a bone fracture. Since the blood is under arterial pressure, it is forced out into the space between the skull and the dura. The hematoma is called epidural because it lies above the dura. This hematoma can become very large and reach a point where it actually compresses the underlying brain. If not treated quickly, it may result in herniation.

The operation is virtually completed with the removal of the bone flap as described earlier. The blood lies immediately below the bone flap so it is easily removed with suction and gentle irrigation with sterile water. Once the blood is removed, a small cut is made in the dura so the surgeon can look at the underlying brain; this is to be sure that there is no blood *below* the dura. Sometimes a subdural hematoma can be missed on a **computed tomography** or **CT** scan if there is an epidural hematoma lying above it. Once the surgeon is sure that there is no blood below the dura, the cut is sutured closed. The bone is replaced as if placing the final piece in a jigsaw puzzle. Small plates and screws or sutures are used to fix the bone flap back into place. These screws prevent the bone flap from becoming dislodged until new bone is formed by the skull.

Subdural Hematomas and Contusions

These two distinct injuries are discussed together because they frequently occur at the same time. The presence of contusions and **subdural hematomas** generally indicates a more forceful injury than that which causes an epidural hematoma. Brain contusions lie deep within the brain and the surgeon, upon opening the dura mater, sees a discolored, bruised brain. Some of this brain is essentially a swollen, nonfunctioning pulp that is no longer functional. The swelling of the injured brain puts the surrounding noninjured areas at risk. If the contused areas swell, they can compress the surrounding viable brain, causing further damage to the brain or compression of blood vessels, which can lead to a massive stroke. Not all subdural hematomas and contusions need be removed, only those that are very large or show signs of out-of-control swelling. Often this swelling is not seen until 24 to 48 hours after the initial injury.

Some patients have contusions and subdural hematomas in different areas of the brain. In this situation, the operation is based on the findings of the patient's preoperative neurologic examination. The brain injuries requiring surgical treatment are those causing neurologic symptoms in the patient. For example, if the patient is paralyzed on the right side but the CT scan shows blood on both sides of the brain, the surgeon will open the left side of the head. Remember, the right side of the brain controls the left side of the body, and vice versa. The surgeon must always couple the CT scan with the findings discovered during the neurologic examination.

Once the site of the operation is determined, it proceeds much like the craniotomy previously described. After the bone flap is removed, a large incision is made in the dura mater to expose the underlying brain. There may be blood lying on top of the brain (subdural hematoma) or parts of the brain may be a bloody pulp (contusions). The subdural hematomas are removed with suction devices and gentle irrigation with sterile water (Figure 6-4). Contusions can also be removed with suction, but bleeding from the surrounding healthy brain must be controlled. Such blood vessels are coagulated (i.e., made to stop bleeding) with a device that uses a very low voltage of electric current. When the subdural blood and contusions are removed, the dura mater is sutured closed and the bone flap is replaced. Sometimes the contused brain shows early signs of swelling. When this happens, the surgeon may choose to leave the

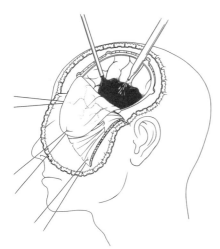

Figure 6-4 Removal of a subdural hematoma. After the bone flap is removed, the dura is opened. This exposes the subdural hematoma present on the surface of the brain. The blood is removed with irrigation and gentle suction such that the brain tissue is not damaged.

bone flap out to provide extra room for the swollen brain. The bone flap is treated with antibiotics and stored in a special freezer; when the patient recovers, the bone flap can be replaced (see discussion of cranioplasty below).

Gunshot Wounds

These injuries are often incredibly devastating and many times irreversibly fatal. The surgeon is often faced with a patient at the point of death and a family demanding that everything be done. Many times doing *everything* for a gunshot wound to the head is to do *nothing*. These patients arrive so seriously injured that any attempt at surgical heroics is destined to fail; even if some survive the operation, they most often die in the postoperative period. The damage caused by bullets entering the brain is directly related to the *speed* of the bullet. As the bullet travels through the brain, it creates incredibly high shearing forces that literally tear the brain apart. Autopsy studies have shown specific sites of brain injury far away from the area the bullet traveled.

With this said, there *are* some patients with penetrating injuries to the head who benefit from operations. Gunshots from low-caliber weapons or those that hit the skull tangentially may create injuries that are amenable to surgical intervention. There have been many studies attempting to predict which patients with gunshot wounds to the head will be salvageable and which will not be. The most important prognostic sign is the level of consciousness at the time of arrival at the emergency department. Generally, patients with a **Glasgow Coma Scale** or **GCS** score of 8 or better have a fair chance of meaningful recovery; for those below GCS 8, the results are exceedingly poor. Results of a CT scan also help determine which patients may benefit from immediate surgery. Often the bullet causes diffuse injuries all over the brain; such a situation will not be helped by surgery. If, however, the damage is localized to a *specific* region, an operation could be helpful.

In general, the surgery is similar to what has been previously described. The craniotomy is performed at the site of the bullet injury. However, the surgical goals are somewhat different in these operations. It is often not possible to remove *all* the bullet fragments. When a bullet hits the skull, it begins to break apart. This causes pieces of bone and bullet fragments to be driven into the brain in many directions (see Figure 3-2). The surgeon must expose the brain and clean up as much as possible without causing further damage. Infection is a concern because with the entry of the bullet, pieces of skin, hair, and dead tissue are driven into the brain. This puts the patient at risk of developing an infection or abscess at the site of injury. By removing the dead tissue and repairing the damaged dura and skin, the surgeon helps decrease the risk of infection. Surgical goals are as follows: remove as much dead brain as possible without damaging surrounding good brain; take out easily accessible bullet, skin, and bone fragments; remove any significant mass lesions (subdural hematomas, contusions, etc.); repair damage to blood vessels; and repair tears in the dura and scalp to help prevent infection.

Many of these patients do poorly despite aggressive surgical and medical treatment. Sometimes there is simply too much damage to repair. Those who survive often need a number of operations to optimize their outcome. Gunshot and other missile injuries to the brain are among the most damaging of all head injuries; they carry an extremely high mortality rate, and those patients who survive are usually left with significant impairments.

DECOMPRESSIVE CRANIOTOMY

Some injuries lie too deep within the brain to reach. In these cases a procedure known as a decompressive craniotomy can be performed. In this operation, a bone flap is removed and the dura is opened. This frees the swelling brain from the constraints of the overlying rigid skull. Sometimes a portion of the temporal or frontal lobe is also removed to create even more room into which the brain can swell. The front portion of these lobes can be removed safely with a *very* low risk of causing a neurologic deficit. This procedure is generally needed if signs of severely raised **intracranial pressure** or **ICP** are present.

CRANIOPLASTY

Cranioplasty refers to an operative procedure in which the bone flap is put back in the skull. This operation is typically performed when the patient has recovered to a certain degree from the initial injury. Hence, this is a relatively good news event for a head injury patient. Further, many think of the skull defect as something unappealing and want the look of their old head back; this indicates a return of cognitive function, also a good sign of recovery.

The operation is performed by reopening the incision from the first craniotomy and freeing up the edges around the skull defect. The bone flap is put back into place and attached with plates and screws or special sutures. A cranioplasty is really the part of the craniotomy that was not performed at the original operation. Sometimes the bone flap does not fit properly due to changes in the skull. In these cases a synthetic bone flap is created from wire mesh, special polymers, or acrylics. Some patients show improvement in their neurologic status after a cranioplasty; while this has been documented in studies, the reason for the improvement is not clearly understood.

REPAIR OF CEREBROSPINAL FLUID LEAK

Although rarely necessary, sometimes a patient will develop leakage of **cerebrospinal fluid** or **CSF** from the nose or ear. This happens when there is a fracture in the base of the skull and a tear in the dural sac. The CSF passes through the tear in the dura and can work its way through the fracture in the skull. Often, simply elevating the patient's head and ordering bedrest will decrease the flow of CSF enough to seal up the hole and stop the leak; other patients require drainage of CSF with a lumbar puncture to help stop the leak. If these two methods fail, an operation is considered to stop the leak. A special CT scan may be necessary to help find the exact site of the leak; a craniotomy is then performed at this site. Since the fracture is at the skull base, the brain is lifted up and a patch placed over the fracture site. Any tears in the dura are also repaired. In some instances the surgeon will take connective tissue and fat from the patient's leg to use as the patch. Surgical repair of CSF leaks is very successful and usually solves the problem. Occasionally, more than one operation is necessary to stop very large leaks.

CAMINO MONITOR AND VENTRICULOSTOMY

Many head injury patients require monitoring of their ICP. Two general methods are used to measure the ICP in these patients. Both use implanted devices placed in the brain through a small hole made in the skull. Twist drills are used to make the hole in the skull. The device is then passed through this hole into the ventricles, or into the surface of the brain. One of the devices is a **Camino monitor,** a fiberoptic wire inserted into the surface of the brain. This device is then secured in place with a bolt that is screwed into the skull (Figure 6-5). The Camino monitor is connected to a pressure transducer that enables the health care staff to continuously monitor the ICP. The drawback is that while the ICP can be *monitored*, the Camino cannot be used to *treat* the elevated ICP.

The other option used to monitor ICP is a **ventriculostomy.** Its benefit is that it not only measures the ICP but also enables the

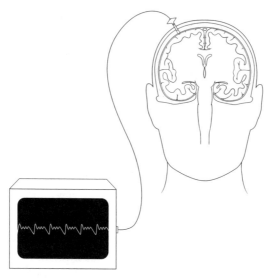

Figure 6-5 Camino monitor. A hole is made in the skull, and a small fiberoptic cable is placed into the surface of the brain. A "bolt" is used, which screws into the skull, to provide stability for the fiberoptic cable. This device is used to continuously monitor intracranial pressure and display this information on a telemetry screen.

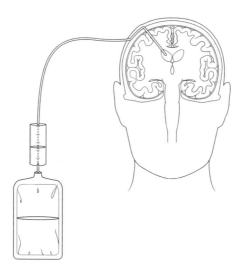

Figure 6-6 Ventriculostomy. A catheter is inserted into the ventricles through a small hole made in the skull. The catheter is "tunneled" underneath the skin, before being connected to the drainage bag, to prevent infection. This device can be used to both continuously monitor the ICP and drain CSF from the ventricles when the ICP is too high.

health care staff to drain CSF from the ventricles when the ICP is elevated. Draining CSF from the brain, when necessary, can help to decrease the ICP. Therefore, the ventriculostomy not only enables continuous ICP measurement, but also allows for the treatment of elevated ICPs. Similar to the Camino monitor, ventriculostomies are passed into the brain through a single small hole made in the skull. Unlike the Camino monitors, however, the small flexible catheters are passed *through* the brain and inserted into the ventricles. Due to the deep location these catheters occupy and the fact that CSF is drained though them, the risk of infection is higher with ventriculostomies. To address this problem, the catheters are tunneled underneath the skin before being connected to the drainage bags. Instead of forming a straight pathway for the bacteria to get into the brain, this maneuver creates a zigzag pathway (Figure 6-6), making it more difficult for bacteria to move along the catheter and into the brain. Patients may also be given antibiotics in an attempt to keep the risk of infection low.

VENTRICULOPERITONEAL SHUNT

Chapter 3 discussed hydrocephalus resulting from traumatic **subarachnoid hemorrhage.** This is infrequent but may develop after head injury. Generally, the more blood that enters the areas containing CSF, the higher the chances for developing hydrocephalus. The **ventriculoperitoneal** or **VP shunt** is a way of bypassing the normal drainage system that has been clogged by the blood. The operation entails placing one end of a tube into the ventricles and running the tube under the skin, while placing the other end into the abdominal cavity. This gives the CSF a way to drain out of the brain into a place where it can be reabsorbed by the body. If this is not done, the fluid will continue to build up until it reaches a critical level and begins to compress vital brain structures. A VP shunt is essentially a permanent ventriculostomy contained inside the body.

ADDITIONAL PROCEDURES AND OPERATIONS

Due to the tremendous forces involved in most accidents, many of these patients have injuries in more than one place in the body. Frequently, they suffer facial fractures or lacerations, broken arms, legs, and necks. Some may even have intra-abdominal or chest injuries. When such multiple injuries are present, treatment becomes more complicated. Cooperation among the neurosurgeons, trauma surgeons, orthopedists, and plastic surgeons is essential to maintain optimal care. The first task is to stabilize the patient and ensure a good airway. Once this is accomplished, the next step is to identify all of the patient's injuries. Care is taken to maintain proper support for the neck, since every patient with a head injury is at high risk of also having a fracture in the neck bones. The trauma patient undergoes a rapid x-ray study and CT scan to identify all the injuries; once identified, they are prioritized. The more life-threatening injuries are addressed first. For example, a patient with an epidural hematoma and a wrist fracture will have a craniotomy to remove the epidural hematoma minutes after arriving at the hospital; the wrist fracture will not be repaired until the patient has recovered from the brain operation. Generally, it is the trauma surgeon and neurosurgeon who decide which injuries are the highest priority. The nonneurosurgical operations associated with these patients are discussed.

Exploratory Laparotomy

When a patient shows signs of internal bleeding, the most common sites are the abdomen and chest. Often the patient is too unstable to go through a battery of x-ray tests, and is taken directly to the operating room for exploratory surgery. The abdomen is opened and the trauma surgeon examines the organs for signs of bleeding. Common causes of internal bleeding are splenic rupture, liver lacerations, and injuries to blood vessels; the general surgeon can repair these and stabilize the patient. Once stabilized, a thorough assessment with x-ray films, CT scans and a complete physical examination can help identify any other injuries.

Thoracotomy

Rarely does a patient bleed so massively that even a short trip to the operating room is impossible. If that is the case, however, it is usually a sign of an injury to one of the major blood vessels in the chest. In this circumstance, the trauma surgeon is forced to open the patient's chest in the emergency department. This is a desperate procedure and is done to stabilize the patient long enough to reach the operating room. As one would suspect, the chances of surviving this procedure are not very good. Luckily, this is relatively uncommon in head injury and more associated with direct penetrating trauma to the chest such as gunshot and stab wounds.

Chest tubes

Many patients involved in motor vehicle accidents suffer both head and chest injuries. This results from the chest hitting the steering wheel and the head impacting the windshield at the time of collision. A fair number of patients sustain rib fractures that may pierce the lung, causing a **pneumothorax.** This occurs when the lung is punctured, and air escapes into the space between the inside of the chest wall and the lung. The air that collects around the outside of the lung can compress the lung and sometimes even the heart. This compression can be so severe as to prevent the lung and heart from functioning and can be fatal. A tube is inserted into this space around the lung that will release the air and allow the lung to re-expand. Hopefully, in a few days, the hole in the lung will seal over and the chest tube can be removed.

Treating Fractures

There is virtually no bone in the body that has not been broken in trauma. Most fractures are considered to be secondary problems in severe head injuries. Two notable exceptions are cervical spine fractures and open extremity fractures. **Cervical spine** injuries are extremely dangerous because they can cause damage to the cervical spinal cord, leaving the patient paralyzed. Many times the patient is placed in cervical traction tongs to stabilize the neck. These tongs attach directly to the skull with pins and hold the neck in a fixed position, which will prevent damage to the underlying spinal cord. Placement of the pins can be difficult if there is a head injury, especially if the patient requires an operation. Patients with spine fractures may need an operation to fix the fractures and prevent spinal cord injury. In most cases these operations can be done after the patient has recovered from the head injury. Some cases require fixation but do not need an operation. These patients are placed in a halo vest, which is a jacket attached to cervical traction tongs. The halo vest does the same thing for a broken neck that a cast does for a broken arm.

Open fractures present a problem for both the orthopedist and the neurosurgeon. An open fracture is a broken bone that lacerates the skin above the fracture. Open fractures are highly susceptible to infection if not cleaned and repaired promptly. Neurosurgeons are very reluctant to allow patients with a head injury to be placed under general anesthesia because, once put to sleep, there is no way to monitor the patient's neurologic status. For this reason, head injury patients who must undergo nonneurosurgical operations generally require insertion of an ICP monitor prior to the operation so the neurosurgeon has a way of monitoring what is going on inside the head. If there is any sign of a problem, the surgery is stopped and the general anesthetic discontinued. The patient is then examined and most probably has a CT scan performed right away.

•————— COMMONLY ASKED QUESTIONS —————•

What are the goals of surgery?

The goals of surgery in head injury patients are to remove any compression on the brain, remove large blood clots and stop the source of the bleeding, decrease elevated ICP (thus improving blood flow to the injured brain), and clean any wounds that could lead to infection within the brain. Compression of normal brain tissue that was not injured at the time of the injury can lead to further damage and loss of function. Blood clots can continue to enlarge and also push on normal portions of the brain, and infections can lead to additional damage. Elevated ICPs can impede the blood flow to the brain, which can lead to strokes and brain cell death. Further, focal compression of the brain and increased ICPs can push the brain up against the brain stem (i.e., the life control center). This, in effect, strangles the brain stem and can rapidly lead to the patient's death. This is called herniation. Therefore most surgery in patients with such injuries is more a necessity than an option, often occurring as an emergency.

Will surgery help?

Injuries that result in the development of mass lesions may be improved with surgery. Mass lesions are types of damage that form a mass in the brain, pushing on the surrounding nondamaged areas, thus causing further damage and increased ICP. Mass lesions can include a bruise within the brain tissue (intracerebral contusion), blood clots outside of the brain's protective covering (epidural hematoma), or a blood clot on the surface of the brain (subdural hematoma). During the operation the blood clot or damaged brain is removed, which takes pressure off the brain, and any bleeding from the blood vessels is stopped.

Patients with large skull fractures that have portions of the broken skull driven into the brain are also taken to the operating room. The bone fragments within the brain are removed, as are any portions of irreversibly damaged brain, and the protective covering of the brain (dura) is then closed. Skull fractures where no fragments have penetrated the brain are usually not operated on, since the fracture will heal on its own. Patients with gunshot wounds to the head are operated on if there are bone fragments within the brain or if there is a large blood clot.

While operations can be beneficial to patients with mass lesions or foreign bodies within the brain, patients with more widespread damage throughout the brain usually do not benefit from an operation. Widespread, nonlocalized injuries, such as shear injuries, or those in which overwhelming damage occurred at the time of the injury, do not benefit from surgery. In the case of shear injury, where the microscopic connections within the brain have been torn apart, there is no way to repair such an injury; there is no target to remove or repair. With patients who suffer devastating injury at the time of the accident, too much damage has already occurred and little can be done for them. Removal of all or even a majority of the damaged brain could result in further brain damage because there is no way to tell for certain if a diffusely damaged area is irreversibly injured. Attempts at removal of this tissue may result in the removal of healthy brain or areas that may have recovered given a chance. The end result could potentially be more loss of function from the operation than if the procedure had not been performed.

Only those with a fair amount of normal brain function truly benefit from surgery; once the brain is irreversibly damaged, it does not grow back. The goal of surgery is often to prevent further damage, to protect the portions of the brain that were not injured, and hopefully to preserve maximum function. Obviously, there are exceptions to this general concept; patients who have widespread damage restricted to one lobe, particularly the temporal or frontal lobe, may benefit from a partial removal of the injured lobe. This is especially true when a damaged area or lobe is exerting a mass effect on the surrounding normal brain, thus causing further damage to areas of the brain that were not injured at the time of the accident.

Another factor in considering surgery is the location of the damage. There are certain areas deep within the brain that are vital for survival, such as the brain stem and thalamus, locations which, if operated on to remove a blood clot or bruise, could result in extensive damage to the patient. In these instances, where the injury is located deep within the brain, it is usually best not to operate. Hopefully, injuries located in these critical areas will resolve with time and intensive medical management. Indeed, in one study it was found that only 37% of the patients with severe injury required surgery.[1]

When do the risks outweigh the benefits?

Anytime surgery is being contemplated the risks must be weighed against the benefits. Ultimately, the preservation of *function* is the goal of all the treatments initiated for these patients. If the risks outweigh the benefits of surgery, the operation will not be performed, since the procedure may do the patient more harm than good. This is true for patients who have bruises deep within the brain in vital areas, such as the thalamus and brain stem. Due to the multitude of connections and important functions that these structures perform, surgery in these locations is too dangerous. In these instances, the risks usually outweigh the benefits and nonsurgical management is selected. The same may be true for bruises located in the speech area (usually on the left side of the brain) and in the motor area (part of the brain that is responsible for moving the arms and legs). Attempts at removal of bruises (i.e., contusions) in these areas may result in permanent loss of speech or movement function.

It is this consideration for the patient and the likely outcomes that the surgeon must weigh when trying to decide if surgery will be beneficial. There is a subtle but important difference between saving a patient's life and providing an opportunity for the patient to have a meaningful, functional recovery. While it may be possible to save a patient's life, that "life" may be one in which the patient is completely vegetative, often in a nursing home. Most people do not want such a situation for themselves or their family members, which is why the surgeon consults with the family members to discuss the potential risks and benefits of any procedure. The surgeon provides the medical knowledge and experience, while the family members can express what they think the patient would want. To some, life is the most important point, regardless of the patient's ability to function, while others feel that it is the *quality* of life that is most important. Only the patient (either by prior discussions or by a living will) and the family can bring these aspects to light and each individual has different viewpoints on this issue. Some feel that every chance of recovery should be provided to the patient, while others feel that unless there is a good chance for a meaningful recovery, the operation should not be performed. Such decisions as to whether a particular operation should be performed are *equally* based on the experiences of the surgeon and the family members' wishes.

What happens to the blood in the patient's head if no surgery is performed?

The blood inside the head resulting from an injury is broken down by the body. Chapter 3 explained that swelling in the brain results from the body sending special substances to the brain to repair damage. These special cells and chemicals attack the blood and break it down into its component parts. These breakdown products are easier for the body to deal with and they are absorbed by special cells. These cells re-enter the blood vessels in the brain and carry off the blood products to the rest of the body where they are further processed and eventually excreted.

Sometimes a small amount of blood is not able to be broken down by the body. This blood may calcify and form a hard rock-like substance. This does not have any harmful affects on the brain and nothing more needs to be done.

Will the blood in the brain cause more brain damage?

There are various types of brain damage that can occur in head injuries. Some of these injuries require immediate surgery, while in other types of injury it may be safer for the patient to closely watch the damaged area rather than perform surgery. A certain amount of blood is often a component of such nonsurgical injuries, such as small or deeply located contusions. While blood inside of the blood vessels is good, blood that has escaped the blood vessels as a result of injury is not. The escaped blood can act as an irritant to the surrounding blood vessels. This irritation can lead to spasm in these vessels, a condition called vasospasm. Severe vasospasm can constrict the blood vessels such that the normal blood flow to the brain is compromised. This can lead to further brain damage and strokes. This is particularly a problem in patients who have a large amount of subarachnoid hemorrhage. The risk of vasospasm appears to correlate somewhat with the amount of blood that has escaped from injured blood vessels. The small amount of blood typically present in smaller contusions does not usually cause a significant problem and, with time, will be reabsorbed by the brain.

Is the bone flap replaced at the time of surgery? If not, what happens later?

Various operations can be performed in head injury patients. The operation performed depends on the type of injury. Most operations for head injury involve a procedure called a craniotomy. During this procedure a bone flap is made with a special drill and removed to allow access to the injured areas within the brain. Following the completion of the surgery within the brain, such as removing a blood clot or contusion, the dura (the protective sac that encases the brain) is usually closed. This helps to cover and protect the brain tissue. The bone flap is replaced and secured in place with either thick suture, wire, or small metal brackets. The muscles and skin, which cover the skull, are closed with sutures or surgical staples.

In some instances, the surgeon may decide not to replace the bone flap when the procedure within the brain is completed. Brain swelling may be such that in order to replace the bone flap, the underlying brain would have to be compressed; this can lead to further brain injury and loss of function. Although a large amount of swelling may not be present at the time of the surgery, the surgeon may still elect to keep the bone flap out if future swelling is anticipated.

As the brain begins to swell in response to the injury, it compresses areas that were not damaged at the time of injury. The ICP also increases, which begins to impede the normal blood flow to the brain from the heart. These two results are potentially harmful if the skull is completely intact. In an attempt to circumvent the compression and elevated ICP, the bone flap may be left out at the time of surgery. This is done in the hope that, by providing more room for the brain to expand, the more crucial internal brain structures, such as the brain stem, will be preserved. Although the bone flap may be left out, the skin and muscles are closed in order to protect the brain from infection.

A drawback to leaving the bone flap out is that the underlying brain remains unprotected from any type of impact. Therefore, the health care staff must be very careful not to place any pressure on that side of the head. Further, if the ICP gets very high despite having the bone flap out, the brain can get pushed out of the opening (i.e., the large hole where the bone flap was) in the skull. In situations where this occurs the amount of brain "pushed out" of this opening can be extensive, leading to severe damage to that area.

Those who survive and recover after the injury can have the opening in the skull repaired; these patients typically have a sunken or indented area where the bone flap was removed. In order to fill in this area, as well as provide protection for the brain against any future impact, another operation is typically performed 3 to 6 months after the injury (although the actual time depends on individual circumstances). Often the patient's original bone flap can be replaced. At the time of the initial operation, the bone flap can be frozen and stored, and later be thawed and replaced in the patient's skull. In cases in which the original bone flap is not suitable, synthetic materials may be used to repair the skull defect. This is done in such a way as to approximate the shape of the original bone flap. In addition to providing cosmesis (i.e., making the patient's head look normal), the materials used are also hard enough to protect the underlying brain.

What is a lumbar puncture and what will it tell you?

A lumbar puncture, also called a spinal tap, is a test in which a physician takes a sample of CSF. As already discussed, CSF is the fluid that baths the brain and spinal cord. This fluid can be collected by inserting a needle in the lower back. There is very little risk of damage to the spinal cord because the needle is inserted into the sac surrounding the spinal cord at a level below the end of the spinal cord. The fluid is sent to the laboratory where a variety of tests are run on the fluid. The most common reason for doing a spinal tap in a patient with a head injury is to rule out or confirm the presence of meningitis, a known complication of head injury, especially when the patient has a CSF leak from the nose or ear. The laboratory routinely measures the amount of protein and glucose in the fluid and also counts the number of red and white blood cells. A small amount of fluid is placed on culture plates to see if any bacteria are present. All these tests provide a profile that should tell the physician if there is an infection **(meningitis)** or not. If these tests show signs of meningitis, the patient requires powerful intravenous antibiotics for at least a week; follow-up lumbar punctures are often performed to make sure the antibiotics are working to defeat the infection.

Another reason for doing a lumbar puncture is to stop a persistent CSF leak. Many times patients with a fracture at the base of the skull also have a tear in the dura covering the brain. This tear in the dura allows the CSF to escape and leak out through the fracture site Most of the time the fracture and tear in the dura will seal up. Occasionally, the leak persists and the longer the leak continues, the higher the risk for developing meningitis. A lumbar puncture may help stop a leak by decreasing the CSF pressure within the brain, giving the dural hole time to close. After removing the fluid, the patient's head is elevated, which also helps to decrease the CSF pressure. In essence, the lumbar puncture and head elevation help decrease the flow through the tear in the dura and help seal it off; this usually works but additional lumbar punctures may be needed to close the leak.

Why is there so much blood in the ventriculostomy?

Some patients may have blood in the ventricles as a result of the injury. Usually patients do not continue to bleed into the ventricles after the injury. The blood clot, however, remains in the ventricles until it dissolves. A ventriculostomy may be necessary to drain off CSF until the normal CSF pathway within the ventricles is reopened as the blood clot dissolves. The CSF drained off by the ventriculostomy remains bloody until the blood clot completely dissolves. In other words, the continued presence of blood-tinged CSF in the fluid drained off by the ventriculostomy does not necessarily mean that the patient is continuing to bleed into the ventricles. Typically the CSF is more bloody initially and then slowly begins to clear as the ventricular clot dissolves. These patients are also followed with serial CT scans to make sure that no new bleeding has occurred.

Why is dye injected into the ventriculostomy?

A ventriculostomy is a catheter inserted into the ventricles (fluid-filled spaces within the brain) to drain off CSF. These catheters may be placed for various reasons, one of which is to treat hydrocephalus. Hydrocephalus is a condition in which the normal CSF pathway is obstructed, resulting in CSF buildup within the ventricles. In the normal pathway, which begins after the CSF is made within the ventricles, the CSF typically flows through the ventricles and then out of the brain down around the spinal cord. The CSF then percolates back up onto the surface of the brain where it is normally absorbed into the bloodstream. Hydrocephalus can result from an obstruction within the ventricles themselves or at the site where the CSF is absorbed into the bloodstream on the surface of the brain.

A patient's clinical course may suggest that the patient has recovered from this condition and no longer requires the ventriculostomy. Before the ventriculostomy is removed, the health care team may want to check to see if the normal CSF pathway between the ventricles and the space around the spinal cord has been re-established. To investigate this possibility, dye, usually dark blue, is injected into the ventriculostomy. This will dye the CSF in the ventricles blue. After a certain period of time, a lumbar puncture is performed. During this procedure CSF is removed from the area around the lower spinal cord. If the CSF obtained is blue, it indicates that the CSF was able to pass from the ventricles out the normal CSF pathways and down around the spinal cord. Such a determination suggests that the normal CSF pathways are intact, although it does not say anything about the CSF absorption mechanism on the surface of the brain, and the ventriculostomy can likely be removed. Patients may, however, redevelop hydrocephalus if the CSF absorptive mechanism on the surface of the brain is occluded (which can occur secondary to blood). In those patients who have hydrocephalus but appear to have re-established the normal CSF pathway from the ventricles to the area around the spinal cord (i.e., those in which the lumbar puncture obtained blue CSF), lumbar punctures can temporarily be used to control the CSF build-up. This may be all that is necessary to control the situation until the normal CSF absorptive mechanism is re-established on the surface of the brain (i.e., when the blood dissolves). Those patients who do not recover may require a VP shunt.

Do the holes from the ventriculostomy close up? Will they cause problems later if they don't?

A ventriculostomy is a procedure in which a small catheter is passed through the brain tissue and inserted into the ventricles. As part of this procedure, a simple twist drill is used to make a small hole in the skull to allow passage of the catheter. The size of the hole made is roughly the size of a thumbtack head. These holes eventually close up on their own as new bone is formed within the skull. Because these holes are relatively small, they usually do not cause any problems. One potential problem, which is fairly uncommon, is the risk of infection. If CSF leaks out of these holes and out through the skin, there is a risk of the patient developing meningitis. Fortunately, this is relatively uncommon, particularly in patients who no longer have elevated ICPs.

How long does a VP shunt last? Does it ever get replaced or taken out?

VP shunts are placed as a treatment for hydrocephalus. These devices are very good at fixing the problem but are very delicate. Like all man-made devices they can break, become clogged, or simply wear out. Another problem with any device implanted into a human being is the risk of infection. Shunt malfunctions and infections usually are recognized because the patient becomes sick.

Generally, patients will develop headache, drowsiness, vomiting and may even show signs of seizures or coma. Patients with a shunt infection may or may not also develop fever and chills. In the case of malfunction, the shunt must be either repaired or replaced in the operating room. Shunt infections are a little more problematic. The infected shunt must be removed but a new one cannot be put in immediately because of the risk of infecting the new shunt from the patient's active infection. If the surgeon were to take out the infected shunt and immediately replace it with a new one, the new shunt system could become infected. In the case of infection, the abdominal end of the shunt is taken out of the abdomen and hooked up to a bag. The infected shunt drains into the bag while the patient is in the hospital receiving intravenous antibiotics. When the infection has been killed by the antibiotics, the entire shunt is removed and a new shunt system is implanted.

There is no set time limit to a shunt system. Some last for many years and never have a problem. These are simply left in place.

How does a VP shunt know how much to drain?

VP shunts are designed to drain CSF out of the ventricles in patients with hydrocephalus and place it into the abdominal cavity where it is then absorbed by the body. These systems are composed of a catheter that is placed in the ventricles, another catheter that runs underneath the skin and into the abdominal cavity (i.e., the peritoneum), and a pressure valve that connects these two catheters. The secret to proper CSF drainage lies in the VP shunt valve. These valves are one-way valves that only allow CSF to drain out of the head (i.e., not back into the head). Further, they are pressure valves, such that CSF only drains out of the ventricles when the pressure in the head is above a certain value. In other words, low pressure valves automatically drain CSF at lower pressures than higher pressure valves. There are a variety of pressure settings available. There are many variables that affect the decision of which valve to choose, but the surgeon customizes the choice to meet the particular needs of the patient.

If there is no external CSF leak, can the patient still have an internal CSF leak that cannot be detected?

CSF leakage is typically due to a skull fracture, which can occur anywhere on the skull. The sharp edges of the fractured bone may tear the dura and cause a CSF leak. The CSF escapes from the brain and, due to gravity, runs along the base of the skull. Depending on the configuration of the fracture, the CSF leaks out of the skull if there is a large enough "hole" available. The presence of a CSF leak is easily identified when there is clear fluid (i.e., CSF) leaking from the nose or ears (external drainage). Other CSF leaks can be more difficult to identify; this is true when the CSF drainage is internal.

For example, CSF can drain into the back of the throat, into the inner ear, or directly into air spaces located within the skull. These internal CSF leaks can be much more difficult to identify, so much so that some may go completely unnoticed. Patients who are leaking CSF into the back of the throat may notice a continuous salty taste in the back of the mouth or something that resembles a continuous postnasal drip; inner ear CSF drainage may lead to decreased hearing in the affected ear. When there is a suspicion of such a leak, CT scans may be obtained in an attempt to find it. The use of dyes injected into the CSF space can also be used to help locate these leaks. Patients who have undetected internal CSF leaks are at risk for repeated bouts of meningitis.

How do you repair a CSF leak?

Most traumatic CSF leaks can initially be treated without surgery. These nonsurgical techniques are used first since most will close without surgery. One nonsurgical method is to elevate the patient's head. The head is elevated anywhere from 30 to 60 degrees in an effort to decrease the amount of CSF leaking from the abnormal pathway; gravity tends to pull the CSF down out of the head and into the space around the spinal cord. The CSF volume within the head is thus decreased, which limits the amount of leakage. Serial lumbar punctures are a more aggressive method to accomplish the same thing. By removing large amounts of CSF from the space around the spinal cord, the overall CSF volume is decreased. This is possible because the CSF spaces in the brain are connected to the space around the spinal cord. The result is that there is less CSF in the head that can leak out through the tear in the dura; by reducing the leakage the tissue in this area is able to heal and close the opening. If these nonsurgical measures are not successful, surgery may be necessary.

In order to surgically repair a CSF leak, the source of the leak must first be located. This can be the most difficult step, especially in patients who have multiple fractures along the base of the skull or those who leak the CSF internally into the back of the throat or inner ear. Among the methods used to locate these leaks, most involve the injection of a dye into the CSF space; in some instances radiographic images, such as a **magnetic resonance imaging** or **MRI** study or **CT scan,** are then taken to pinpoint the source of the problem.

Once the site of the leak is located, surgery can be performed if necessary to repair the damage. A **craniotomy** is performed to expose the dura (the protective covering around the brain). The dura is inspected and any small tears are closed with suture. However, the dural injury may be so extensive that this may not be possible, as is often the case in patients with multiple fractures along the base of the skull. In these instances, where there are many large tears, additional tissue must be used to patch the dura closed. The thin layer of tissue that covers the skull, called the pericranium, is often used to repair these tears. A similar tissue, located in the side of the thigh, can also be used to patch these dural tears. Once the dura is repaired, the bone flap is replaced and the skin is closed. Any fractures of the skull are also repaired as necessary.

What are the complications of a CSF leak?

Fortunately, the majority of CSF leaks secondary to head injury heal by themselves without any surgical intervention. The major risk for any CSF leak is infection. The presence of an external CSF leak indicates there is an abnormal communication or pathway between the space around the brain and the skin. While CSF can escape through this passageway, even more important, bacteria can travel from the skin into the space around the brain. This can lead to **meningitis,** which is a serious infection of the brain. It is for this reason that some patients receive antibiotics if a CSF leak is detected. This is done in an attempt to reduce the risk of developing meningitis before the leak closes. Patients who have persistent CSF leaks, particularly those in which the site of the leak is difficult to identify, can have repeated bouts of meningitis. To prevent this, patients with persistent CSF leakage often require surgical intervention to repair the leak. Surgery is usually successful in repairing these abnormalities that do not heal by themselves.

In addition to the risk of infection, CSF leakage can also cause headaches, nausea, and vomiting. This is especially true when the patient is in an upright position or those in which the leak is very large. In general, the more CSF that leaks out of the head, the worse these symptoms tend to be. These symptoms sometimes improve with the administration of intravenous fluids.

When will other body injuries be fixed? Are these life threatening?

Patients with head injury often have additional injuries as a result of the accident. These injuries are addressed according to their severity and the overall risk each poses to the patient. This is why many different specialists are typically involved in the comprehensive management of these patients. Each specialty team assesses the patient and the group then decides which injuries pose the greatest threat to the patient's well-being. Life-threatening injuries, such as massive blood loss, extensive internal organ damage, and poor oxygen intake, are treated immediately. The treatment of other non–life-threatening injuries, such as broken bones and facial fractures, are typically definitively treated when the patient is medically stable. Nonsurgical management is utilized in treating these injuries until the patient's condition improves. Repair of non–life-threatening injuries may also be delayed in patients who have severe head injuries. Patients at risk for **herniation,** including those with elevated ICPs or large brain contusions, are given an opportunity to recover from the brain injury before surgery is performed to repair nonlife-threatening injuries. This delay is designed to protect the patient from any further potential damage while the brain's condition is unstable.

Will the bullet be removed? What about the bullet fragments?

Patients with gunshot wounds to the head typically suffer extremely serious brain injuries. In fact, most patients with this type of injury do not survive, particularly those in which the bullet traveled through both sides of the brain. Although the bullet causes direct tearing as it moves through the brain, the majority of the damage relates to the forces transferred from the speeding bullet to the brain. This occurs instantaneously when the bullet quickly moves through the brain. Unfortunately, very little can be done for the resulting damage.

Surgery is sometimes performed on these patients if a large blood clot is present. This is done when it is thought that the patient's condition may improve on removal of the blood clot. Surgery may also be performed in patients who show signs that they may survive the injury and actually improve. In this case the purpose of the procedure is to close the dura and clean the wounds in an attempt to decrease the risk of infection. Bullet fragments, bone fragments, and the bullet itself, if it is easily identified at the time of the surgery, are removed during the operation as well. It is not imperative, however, to remove the bullet in most patients. Given this, most neurosurgeons are reluctant to potentially cause further damage while searching through the brain tissue for the bullet. As is true when considering any surgical procedure, the option of surgery is elected when it is thought that the procedure will benefit the patient.

REFERENCE

1. Marshall LF, Gautille T, Klauber MR, et al. The outcome of severe closed head injury. J Neurosurg 75:S28-S36, 1991.

CHAPTER

7

$\infty\!\!\!\infty\cdot\!\infty\!\!\!\infty$

The Intensive Care Setting: Demystifying the Wires, Tubes, and Beeping Machines

Most patients with moderate to severe head injury are admitted to the **intensive care unit** or **ICU** in the hospital. While the ICU setting can be intimidating to family members unfamiliar with this environment, it is here that the patient receives the most comprehensive and focused medical care. At first glance family members can often be overwhelmed by the multitude of wires, tubes, and "beeping" machines going into, out of, and surrounding the patient (Figure 7-1).

> **Donna:** It was extremely frightening to see my sister hooked up to all the monitors. It made me realize how serious it was. I was hopeful the technology would make a difference, but I still questioned whether she was going to be okay, what she was going to be like if she came out of this.
>
> Sharon was in an induced coma for an experimental treatment study. She was also on a ventilator and had a broken rib and punctured lung. Even though she was in a coma, we talked to her all of

the time, just in case she could hear us. I read to her and many times would start crying, because a lot of what we read were her cards. She had tons of cards from friends and loved ones who wrote such wonderful things. I'd stop reading them and compose myself and then continue to read. Sometimes I wish I would have taken a picture or videotaped the room while she was in there, but I couldn't bring myself to do it . . . I could visit for 10 minutes and most of the time I just went in there and asked the nurse questions. I was constantly asking, "What's going on, how's the pressure in her brain and the blood pressure?"

In an attempt to make sense of this medical management chaos, some general definitions and explanations of all this equipment follow.

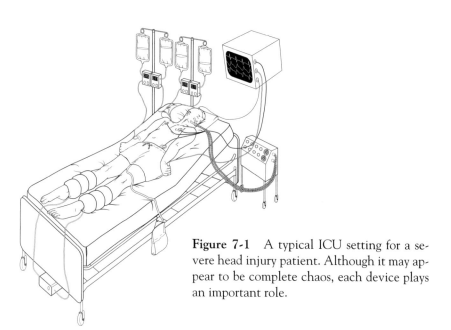

Figure 7-1 A typical ICU setting for a severe head injury patient. Although it may appear to be complete chaos, each device plays an important role.

THE VENTILATOR (BREATHING MACHINE) AND THE TUBE

As discussed earlier, most patients suffer some degree of unconsciousness as a consequence of their head injury. Those who are deeply unconscious may have difficulty breathing, a situation that can lead to death if untreated. Therefore, many patients with head injury have a tube called an **endotracheal tube** placed through their mouth and into their main breathing passageway ("windpipe" or **trachea**); when such a tube is in place, patients are said to be **intubated.** The endotracheal tube helps to protect the airway and enables the health care staff to assist the patient breathe appropriately. The machine that assists the patient's breathing is called a **ventilator** or "respirator" (Figure 7-2). The ventilator is an incredibly useful machine that can control how much oxygen the patient receives, how deep each breath is, and how fast the patient breathes; these different settings enable the health care team to optimize the patient's care.

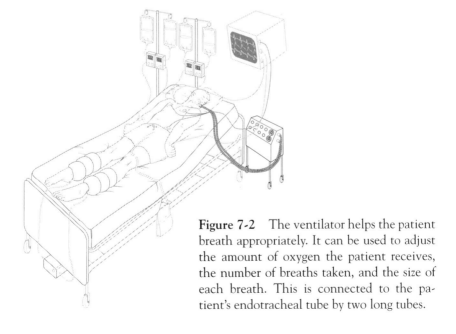

Figure 7-2   The ventilator helps the patient breath appropriately. It can be used to adjust the amount of oxygen the patient receives, the number of breaths taken, and the size of each breath. This is connected to the patient's endotracheal tube by two long tubes.

Due to incidents that have been reported in the newspapers and on television, some people may have some misconceptions regarding ventilator usage. The term "life support" comes up within this context, which, unfortunately, has taken on a negative connotation. In effect, all the medical care provided after the accident is "life support" because it is directed at saving the patient's life. Although a patient may be intubated and placed on a ventilator, this is by no means a permanent situation; many improve while on the ventilator and can subsequently have the breathing tube removed called extubation. Still others, who remain to a certain degree unconscious and therefore have difficulty keeping their airway open, may have a tube placed through the neck into the windpipe (a tracheostomy). Even though unconscious, these patients often do not require ventilator assistance for extended periods of time; the ventilator merely assists until the normal breathing patterns return. In patients who do not recover or in whom the neurologic injury is so devastating that a meaningful recovery is unlikely, the family can request that the ventilator be discontinued.

THE "LINES OF SPAGHETTI"

One of the most striking sights in the neurosurgical ICU rooms is the large number of small plastic tubes present. Intertwined and often multicolored, they go into and out of the patient, resembling a multicolored spaghetti dish. Called **intravenous lines** or **IVs,** they deliver necessary medications and fluids (Figure 7-3). These lines in the patient's veins must be changed periodically to a different location in an attempt to prevent infection.

While some of the small tubes (i.e., intravenous lines) are used for medications and fluids, others monitor important aspects of the patient's condition. An **arterial line** is a catheter (i.e., tube) inserted into an artery (usually in the wrist) to continuously monitor blood pressure, enabling the health care staff to immediately detect and treat any abnormalities. This is important as a low blood pressure can result in less blood getting to the brain, while elevated

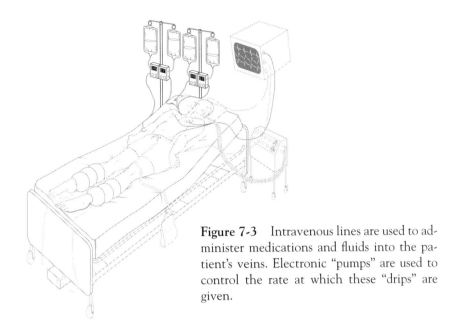

Figure 7-3   Intravenous lines are used to administer medications and fluids into the patient's veins. Electronic "pumps" are used to control the rate at which these "drips" are given.

blood pressures can enlarge existing blood clots. Another specialized catheter, inserted into a large vein in the neck, may be used to monitor heart function and the overall fluid status of the patient. This is called a **Swan-Ganz catheter.**

Other tubes or catheters that may be required include the **Foley catheter,** a smooth rubber catheter inserted into the patient's bladder, that provides precise measurement (on an hourly basis) of the urine volume produced by the kidneys, information useful in determining how well the kidneys are functioning; the **nasogastric** or **NG tube,** which is inserted through the nose or mouth and down the swallowing tube **(esophagus)** into the stomach, that enables the health care staff to administer medications *directly* into the stomach (the NG tube can also be used to suction out the stomach contents, which may be necessary if the stomach and intestines are not working properly), and the **Dobhoff tube,** which is smaller and more flexible than the NG tube. This is also inserted into the stomach through the mouth or nose and is typically used to provide nu-

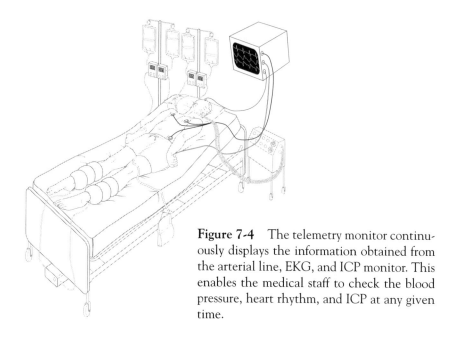

Figure 7-4 The telemetry monitor continuously displays the information obtained from the arterial line, EKG, and ICP monitor. This enables the medical staff to check the blood pressure, heart rhythm, and ICP at any given time.

trition to patients who are unable to eat (it can also be used to administer certain medications).

In addition to these multiple lines of "spaghetti," most patients also have wires connected to their chest. These are connected to little "stickers" on the patient's skin called **EKG leads.** These continuously monitor the heart's electrical activity and rhythm. This information, displayed on a **telemetry monitor** (Figure 7-4) at the bedside, detects any abnormal heart rhythms or electrical activity.

BRAIN PRESSURE MONITORING AND TREATMENT

A major problem that occurs with head injury is brain swelling or **cerebral edema.** Much the way a knee swells up after a fall, the brain also swells in response to head injury, and, as with a knee, eventually the swelling (edema) resolves. One essential key in the treatment of these patients is to keep brain swelling to a minimum, since too much swelling can choke the brain, decreasing its blood supply. This can lead to devastating strokes and death.

Depending on the severity of the head injury, it may be necessary to directly monitor the brain pressure (**intracranial pressure** or **ICP**). This can be continuously measured, as the blood pressure is with an arterial line, in two different ways. Both methods are performed at the bedside in the ICU. One method involves the placement of a catheter into the deep, fluid-filled spaces within the brain, the **ventricles,** through a small hole made in the skull. This enables continuous measurements of the ICP. When the pressure is too high, fluid can be drained from the ventricles, thereby decreasing the ICP directly. This is called a **ventriculostomy.** The second method is used when the fluid-filled spaces are too small to get a catheter inside. In this case, a special fiber can be placed into the surface of the brain. This fiber, called a **Camino monitor,** can continuously measure the ICP, but does not allow drainage of the fluid-filled spaces if the pressure is too high.

Sarah: I stayed with Jim around the clock the whole first week. When they told me that he was coming out of the coma, that they were taking away the coma-inducing drugs, I was naturally very anxious and eager. But it took longer than I expected for the drugs to wear off. He woke up gradually, not like waking up in the morning. It was frightening and hard to see my husband that way. His head was totally bandaged and the monitor was sticking out of it. He was moving a lot, not saying anything, surrounded and enveloped by all the monitors and wires. The nurses did a great job explaining what all the monitors were for.

Patients with severe head injuries often have elevated ICP, which, as was discussed before, is detrimental since it tends to decrease the blood supply to the brain. If left uncontrolled, the pressure can snowball, steadily increasing and leading to death of the patient. In those instances, when drainage of the fluid-filled spaces is not possible or is insufficient to keep the ICPs under control, other treatments are initiated. Patients with dangerously elevated ICPs as a result of restlessness or agitation may be given sedation and medications that artificially paralyze the patient called **paralytics.** When these two medications are given, usually in combination, the patient does not move or respond to any type of stimulus. This combination often helps to control the ICP, as well as help in breathing for a patient with lung damage.

Mannitol, a medication that causes the brain swelling to decrease, typically is given when the ICP is too high. This medication is often effective in temporarily controlling the elevated pressure but it can hurt the patient's kidneys if too much is given. To prevent damage to the kidneys, the patient's blood is drawn regularly to check the electrolytes and **serum osmolarity.** The results of these tests help to guide the physician as to how much and how often the mannitol can be given. Hyperventilation, using the ventilator to increase the patient's rate of breathing, can also temporarily decrease elevated brain pressure.

In certain situations when the ICP cannot be controlled with these interventions, the patient may be given a medication that puts the brain into a very deep "sleep." This artificial coma, termed **pentobarbital coma,** is a last-ditch effort to keep the elevated ICP under control until the brain swelling dissipates. This medication, similar to the combination of sedation and chemical paralysis, works directly on the brain and essentially "turns it off." This is thought to be somewhat protective to the injured brain and may help to control the brain swelling until it begins to resolve on its own. Although not always effective, pentobarbital coma can be a valuable treatment in those patients with uncontrolled brain swelling.

THE MACHINES THAT GO BEEP

As should now be clear, the care of head injuries is very complicated. There are ongoing, continuous measurements of many functions, ranging from breathing to ICP. Most of this information is displayed on an electrical monitor that is often near or above the patient. This telemetry monitor is usually easy to pick out; it is the screen that has all the bouncing line tracings on it. These tracings, which are usually labeled on the screen, display the continuous measurements of the blood pressure, ICP, the electrical heart activity and rate, and the breathing rate. Each individual telemetry monitor, with all its measurements, is also displayed on *one central monitor* in the ICU. Both the central and individual telemetry monitors are extremely useful as they sound an alarm if any of these measurements becomes abnormal. This alerts the medical staff that something is wrong and treatment can then be immediately started to correct the problem.

Another beeping machine is called the **pulse oximeter.** This is often a small rectangular box that displays flashing red or green lights. The amount of oxygen in the patient's blood is measured with this device through a small clamp placed over a finger, earlobe, or toe. The pulse oximeter sounds an alarm if the oxygen content is too low, alerting the medical staff that more oxygen should be given. One drawback to this particular device is that it alarms if the clamp falls off the patient, a not uncommon occurrence, especially if the patient is agitated or restless. The alarm in this particular instance does not mean that anything is wrong, simply that the clamp needs to be replaced on the body.

Finally, the ventilator (the breathing machine) sounds off if any of the tubing in the patient becomes disconnected, indicating that the patient is not getting enough help breathing.

Family members can often be overwhelmed by all the tubes, wires, and alarms, which at times can go off simultaneously. Keep in mind, however, that the medical staff are trained professionals, very familiar with all the alarms, tubes, and wires that can seem to family members like a scene from a science fiction movie. Remember, those devices can spell the difference between life and death.

Ellen: *Steve was hooked up to all kinds of monitors and had a probe or something inserted to measure the brain waves. The first 72 hours are especially critical. It was scary seeing him in that hospital bed. If they hadn't told me that was my son, I would not have recognized* *him because he was so swollen. It was just unbelievable how he looked. My first husband didn't have a mark on him following his accident, but he was hit on the back of the head. And obviously his case was more serious than it appeared.*

COMMONLY ASKED QUESTIONS

How can you monitor the amount of brain swelling?

When the brain swells, there is an increase in the total pressure within the cranial cavity (i.e., the head). Since the skull is a rigid structure any time the brain expands it creates more pressure inside the cranial vault. Picture a balloon inside a glass box. As the balloon is inflated, it pushes against the insides of the box. Eventually the pressure created by the expansion of the balloon is so great that the balloon bursts. Brain swelling is essentially the same thing; the brain expands inside a rigid box and the pressure created is directed back up on the brain. To monitor this pressure monitors are placed inside the ventricles of the brain (ventriculostomy) or just under the skull (Camino monitor). These devices measure the pressure inside the skull. By monitoring the pressure the physician is able to more precisely institute specific therapy.

What is a ventriculostomy or Camino monitor?

These devices are placed inside the head to continuously measure the ICP; knowing this pressure guides the neurosurgeon in making treatment decisions. There are certain drugs (mannitol and sedatives) that can be given to lower the ICP. The Camino monitor and ventriculostomy are similar in that they both measure the pressure inside the head. The Camino monitor is placed within the surface of the brain tissue. This monitor is a fiberoptic cable that measures the pressure inside the head and displays this data on a view box. It is anchored to the skull with a metal clamp called a bolt screwed into the skull; this prevents it from becoming dislodged during routine patient care, such as turning, physical therapy, and bathing.

The ventriculostomy is somewhat more complicated than the

Camino monitor. The ventriculostomy is a long tube placed into the lateral ventricle within the brain. This allows a direct measurement of the pressure inside the brain and also allows the physician to drain off fluid. Removing fluid also helps lower the ICP and provides room for the brain to swell. Because insertion of a ventriculostomy is technically more difficult, and many times the ventricles are too small to get a tube into them, placement of a Camino monitor is often the only option.

How long can a ventriculostomy or Camino monitor stay in?

The major risk in having a ventriculostomy or Camino ICP monitor in place is infection. This risk is higher for a ventriculostomy, which is located deep within the brain's fluid-filled spaces (the ventricles), but it is also present with Camino monitors. Patients with these in place are typically given antibiotics to help prevent infection. Ventriculostomies are usually changed every 7 to 10 days for as long as the patient requires intracranial drainage. Ventriculostomies left in place for longer than 10 days have an increased risk of infection.

Some patients, however, may have very small ventricles (where the ventriculostomy is inserted) secondary to elevated ICPs. In such patients, who still require ICP monitoring and drainage, it may not be possible to change the ventriculostomy as regularly. In this situation, the risk of infection with the ventriculostomy is weighed against the risk of not being able to drain the ventricles and control the elevated ICP. If drainage is not necessary to control the ICP, the ventriculostomy may be removed and replaced with a Camino ICP monitor if monitoring is still necessary. Camino monitors can typically be left in place for longer periods of time, anywhere from 10 to 14 days. Usually, however, these are also changed every 7 to 10 days to keep the risk of infection low.

What are the risks associated with having and placing a ventriculostomy?

The risks regarding the placement of a ventriculostomy include bleeding and damage to normal portions of the brain. Another risk is that the ventriculostomy catheter may not actually get into the ventricles. A ventriculostomy catheter is passed through a small hole made in the skull; it is then passed through the brain into the fluid-filled spaces deep within the center of the brain (i.e., the ventricles). Passage of the catheter can cause bleeding within the brain tissue. A large amount of bleeding may result in damage to the brain and require an emergency operation to remove the blood clot. Fortunately, this risk of bleeding is low. The catheters used are small and flexible and, hence, they usually cause very little damage to the actual brain tissue as they are passed through the brain. The risk of unsuccessful insertion of the catheter into the ventricles relates to the size of these fluid-filled spaces. Patients with large blood clots within the ventricles or those with very high ICP may have very small fluid-filled spaces available for the catheter to be inserted; the smaller the target, the more difficult it is to hit.

The major risk of having a ventriculostomy in place is infection. This risk increases the longer the catheter is left in place. For this reason the ventriculostomies are usually changed every 7 to 10 days if possible. Patients are also typically given antibiotics in an attempt to keep the risk of infection low. The fluid that is drained from the ventriculostomy is also routinely checked for evidence of infection.

An article in the newspaper said that all head injury patients should have an ICP monitor. Why isn't my family member being monitored?

Not every head injury patient needs an ICP monitor. The monitor is used for severe head injury patients (i.e., unconscious, exhibiting posturing responses) where increased ICP is a major concern and for those in whom serial neurologic examinations are not possible (i.e., chemically sedated patients). It should be kept in mind that placing a monitor inside a patient's head is not without risk. The ventriculostomy tube actually passes through the brain and enters the ventricular system. As the tube passes through the brain, there is a small chance it could hit a blood vessel and cause an intracranial hemorrhage, possibly resulting in a stroke. Both the ventricular catheter and Camino monitor have a small but definite risk of infection. An infection in either of these devices can result in meningitis, which can be a life-threatening problem. Fortunately, the risk of causing a hemorrhage or developing an infection is relatively low with these ICP monitoring devices. Even so, these monitors are only used when absolutely necessary. The patient should not be subjected to the risk of monitor insertion if its use will not significantly change treatment.

What is ICP?

ICP is the pressure within the skull and is one important measurement used by the health care staff to assess how healthy or damaged the brain is at any given moment. The ICP is typically measured with a ventriculostomy (a catheter placed deep within the fluid-filled spaces of the brain) or with a Camino monitor (a small fiberoptic cable inserted into the surface of the brain). The brain tends to swell in response to the injuries sustained at the time of the accident. It is this swelling (cerebral edema) that, if not controlled, can lead to further damage to the brain and even to the death of the patient. As the brain swelling increases, the ICP will increase. The increase in ICP is a sign to the health care staff that the brain swelling is continuing and that something must be done to correct this potentially lethal situation. If the ICP increases rapidly, it may suggest that a condition, such as a blood clot or **contusion** (a bruise on the brain), is enlarging. A **computed tomography** or **CT** scan of the brain is usually obtained if this rapid increase in ICP occurs, and surgery may be necessary when a large blood clot or contusion is found.

What is a normal ICP?

A normal ICP for adults is approximately 15 mm Hg (or 150 cm H_2O). The normal ICP for young children is lower because of the way their skull is configured. Although 15 is the *upper* limit of normal, most neurosurgical ICUs do not attempt to lower the ICP until it is 20 to 25 mm Hg (or 200 to 250 cm H_2O). This is because these higher levels seem to be tolerated without side effects. While the treatments for elevated ICP can be effective, those same treatments may have bad side effects if used too aggressively. Therefore most health care staff members elect to withhold treating the ICP until it is greater than 20 to 25.

Also keep in mind that certain factors, such as severe agitation and coughing into the breathing tube (endotracheal tube), can increase the ICP. While the reading on the telemetry screen might show that the ICP is high, it may be elevated, not from the injured brain, but from these other "nonbrain" factors. In these circumstances, treatment is usually not specifically directed at decreasing brain swelling but rather aimed at removing the *cause* of the increased ICP. For example, an agitated patient with an elevated ICP may be given a sedative; this acts to calm the patient down and decrease the ICP.

What is CPP?

Cerebral perfusion pressure or **CCP** is the difference between the blood pressure in the body and the ICP. It helps to think of them as two opposing pressures. The blood pressure in the body, which is due in part to the pressure made by the heart (the **systemic blood pressure**), is trying to get blood and necessary oxygen into the brain. Think of this as the "good pressure." The ICP, which is the pressure in the head and brain, acts to keep blood out of the brain. Think of this as the "bad pressure." The systemic blood pressure must overcome the ICP in order to get the necessary blood to the brain. If the ICP is stronger than the systemic blood pressure, no blood will get into the brain. This results in a massive stroke in the entire brain, a fatal situation.

Most treatment of patients with significant head injury, and resultant elevated ICP, attempts to optimize the CPP. This is done by keeping the ICP low (keeping the "bad" pressure low) and keeping the systemic blood pressure high enough to supply the brain with blood (keeping the "good" pressure high). Studies have suggested (although not yet proven) that keeping the CPP at approximately 70 results in better outcomes for patients with severe head injury.

When the ICP increases, what changes can we expect to see?

A certain response can occur in patients with dangerously elevated ICPs. When the ICP gets high enough to cause compression of the brain stem, the blood pressure can get very high while the heart rate (pulse) gets very low. This response is a sign that the brain stem's function is beginning to be affected by the increased pressures within the brain. If the ICP increases or remains elevated, the compression on the brain stem can lead to irreversible damage. The brain pushes up against the brain stem and, in effect, strangles it of its blood supply. This is called herniation, which results when the life control center (located in the brain stem), which helps control the heart rate, breathing, and blood pressure, becomes damaged from the compression. The heart may stop beating, the blood pressure can drop very low, and breathing may stop. Typically, one or both of the pupils become very dilated when this occurs. Obviously, if the compression against the brain stem is not quickly corrected, it may lead to the patient's death.

How high can the ICP get without causing any injury?

The upper limit of normal ICP in normal people is about 15 mm Hg (or 150 cm H_2O) (as measured by a Camino monitor or ventriculostomy and displayed on the telemetry monitor). As the brain begins to swell in response to the injury, the ICP begins to increase. As it increases, it becomes more and more difficult for the heart to overcome the elevated pressure to get the necessary blood into the brain. The CPP, the difference between the blood pressure and the ICP, is the measurement used to ascertain this relationship. As long as the blood pressure is sufficiently *greater* than the ICP, an adequate blood supply to the brain will be maintained. As the difference between the blood pressure and the ICP decreases, less and less blood gets to the brain. Thus it is really the CPP that is most important. Although it remains to be proven, multiple studies of head injury patients indicate that maintaining a CPP at or slightly above 70 results in better recovery. Most health care teams attempt to keep the ICP at or below 20 to help improve blood flow to the brain in these head injury patients.

The presence of contusions within the brain can complicate matters. Contusions in certain locations within the brain are more likely to put pressure on vital structures (such as the brain stem). An example is a contusion within the **temporal lobe,** which is very close to the brain stem. This situation may be such that the temporal lobe is even closer to the brain stem, because of focal swelling caused by the contusion, increasing the risk of herniation and death. Therefore, to prevent any further encroachment on the brain stem, the ICP may need to be kept lower than in those patients who do not have contusions within the temporal lobe. By keeping the ICP lower, the pressures attempting to push the temporal lobe into the brain stem are decreased. In these circumstances, the health care staff may attempt to keep the ICP less than 15. It should be noted, however, that it may not be possible to keep the ICP at the desired level, particularly in patients with severe injuries. The health care staff will then attempt to keep the ICP as low as possible until the swelling begins to resolve, hopefully before irreversible damage occurs.

Why does the ICP remain high after draining off the CSF?

ICP is common in the more severe head injuries. This can result from either focal damage in the brain or more diffuse-type injuries in which the *entire* brain begins to swell. As the swelling increases, normal parts of the brain, not injured at the time of the accident, are now subjected to increased pressure. These areas can become damaged by the compression resulting from these increased pressures. In addition, the increased ICP acts to impede the normal blood flow to the brain. As the blood flow decreases, the individual brain cells do not get enough oxygen. These cells may die as a result, and, if a large number of these cells die, extensive damage can occur. As more damage occurs, the ICP increases, which further increases the damage within the brain, creating a vicious cycle.

In some cases it may be possible to insert a catheter into the fluid-filled spaces (ventricles) within the brain. This is called a ventriculostomy, which allows for simultaneous ICP measurement and **cerebrospinal fluid** or **CSF** drainage. By decreasing the amount of fluid in the ventricles the ICP may be decreased. The problem is that the amount of fluid in the ventricles is generally small. Increased ICP may compress the ventricles, making the amount of fluid contained within these structures even smaller; hence, it may only be possible to drain very small amounts of CSF with the ventriculostomy. In patients who have a large amount of brain swelling (cerebral edema), drainage of such small amounts of CSF may not decrease the ICP very much. But the problem in head injury is that the *brain* is swelling from the injury, *not the ventricles*; while CSF drainage from the ventricles can sometimes help decrease the ICP, it doesn't do anything for the actual brain swelling. It is more a method used to gain time until the brain swelling begins to decrease.

Can draining the CSF cause damage? Can you drain too much CSF?

CSF may be drained from a patient for several reasons. A lumbar puncture (i.e., a spinal tap) may have to be performed to obtain a CSF sample when the presence of an infection (i.e., meningitis) is suspected. The sample is sent to the laboratory for cultures to see if there are bacteria present in the fluid. This procedure can also give an indication of the ICP in some patients. The amount of CSF that is drained in this instance is relatively small. Larger volumes may be drained if the medical staff is performing the lumbar puncture in an attempt to stop a CSF leak. In general, lumbar punctures (LPs) are low-risk procedures, although some patients may develop a transient headache after it is completed. A lumbar puncture is typically not done in patients who have large focal areas of brain damage that are compressing the adjacent tissue. Drainage of CSF from the space around the spinal cord in this situation could cause herniation. If it is necessary to obtain a CSF sample in this circumstance, the fluid can be obtained from the ventricles themselves.

CSF drainage is also used to help control elevated ICPs in head injury patients. This is typically done with a ventriculostomy catheter. CSF is drained whenever the ICP gets too high. Although small volumes are removed with each drainage, the total amount of CSF removed over the course of a day may be relatively large. As long as the amount of CSF removed with each drainage is small, the risk for damage to the brain is relatively low. This risk increases if large amounts are removed all at once. This can cause bleeding on the surface of the brain, leading to the formation of a **subdural hematoma.** Therefore, the risk of damage relates to the amount of CSF removed with each drainage, not necessarily the total amount drained over the course of a day. There is also a risk of bleeding within the ventricles themselves when the CSF is drained with a ventriculostomy; the risk is fairly low but it can occur. In addition, some patients may become "dependent" on the ventricular drainage when the ventriculostomy catheter must be kept in place for long periods of time. These patients, in which the normal CSF absorption mechanism no longer functions properly, may require a **ventriculoperitoneal shunt.**

Why is the fluid draining from the ventriculostomy a red-brownish color?

Ventriculostomy catheters are inserted into the fluid-filled spaces deep within the brain called the ventricles. These are filled with CSF. Normally, the CSF looks just like water when it is drained from the catheter. However, patients who have blood in the ventricles as a result of the injury will have red-colored (i.e., bloody) CSF. This does not necessarily mean that the patient is bleeding within the ventricles, especially if it is not a new occurrence. The CSF will remain bloody as long as there is a fresh blood clot inside the ventricles. As the blood clot starts to break down, the fluid begins to change to a more brown-yellow color. Gradually, the fluid begins to clear up again as the blood is dissolved. Caution must be used, however, as infected CSF can look brown-yellow. This is why CSF is routinely sent to the laboratory for cultures to determine whether there are any bacteria in the fluid indicating an infection that needs to be treated.

What is the treatment for cerebral edema?

Mannitol is a drug that helps control brain swelling. It acts in a variety of ways to decrease the pressure within the brain. By limiting the leak of water and other body fluids into the brain, the total amount of swelling can be controlled. The edema reaches a peak approximately 48 to 72 hours after the brain injury. If the ICP can be controlled during this critical period, the edema will start to subside on its own and the patient will be out of danger. There are methods to control increased ICP other than mannitol. These include ventriculostomy drainage, **hyperventilation,** surgical decompression, and sedation. None of these methods is a treatment of edema, but rather another way to lower ICP.

What is the purpose of a Swan-Ganz catheter?

A Swan-Ganz or pulmonary artery catheter is a device used to monitor fluid status and heart-lung function. The catheter is placed in a large vein that enters the heart and it is then "floated" through the chambers of the right side of the heart until the tip rests in the **pulmonary artery.** The catheter's tip has a small balloon that can be inflated to measure pressure inside the pulmonary artery. This pressure measurement provides the physician with a **hemodynamic profile** for the patient. Controlling cerebral edema is a big part in helping the patient recover from a brain injury; by knowing the overall fluid status, the physician can treat high ICP more safely and more effectively.

What is a ventilator?

A ventilator (or respirator) is a machine that breathes for or helps the patient breathe. Some patients may be completely dependent on the machine to do all the breathing, while others need only a little help. The ventilator can be used to deliver the number of breaths per minute and the oxygen concentration can also be adjusted. Patients on a ventilator often have arterial blood samples taken to measure the oxygen and carbon dioxide concentrations in their blood; the machine can then be adjusted to alter these concentrations in the blood as necessary.

While the ventilator is effective at moving air in and out of the lungs, the patient's lungs still must do *some* of the work. The oxygen we breathe is filtered by the lungs in a special way to remove oxygen from the air and place it into the blood. The ventilator cannot do this, only the lungs can; therefore, even if the patient is not breathing, the lungs are still doing a lot of the work of respiration.

Some patients can breathe on their own but are too deeply unconscious to protect their airway. This impairment puts patients at risk for aspirating, so the breathing tube is left in to protect the airway. Many times this is only temporary, until the patient wakes up, but sometimes a tracheostomy is needed for longer term airway protection.

How long will the patient be on the ventilator? How do you know when to take the patient off the ventilator?

The length of time a patient is on a ventilator depends on the reason the ventilator was initially necessary. Certain injuries or medical conditions take longer to resolve than others. Head injury patients are often intubated and placed on the ventilator when they arrive at the hospital; patients with more severe injuries are usually unconscious. This depressed level of consciousness may result in poor breathing, which can be dangerous for these patients. Just as the level of awareness is decreased, the normal drive to breathe can also be blunted. Patients in this state, who don't breathe either rapidly enough or deeply enough, may not get adequate oxygen into their blood. The brain needs oxygen to survive, especially in the setting of a brain injury.

As protection, these patients are intubated and placed on the ventilator to make sure they get enough oxygen. Similarly, the ventilator can breathe for those patients who are "too asleep" to breathe, making sure that the required number of breaths are taken each minute. This helps to keep the carbon dioxide levels in the blood normal. High carbon dioxide levels, which can occur if the patient does not breathe rapidly enough, can increase any brain swelling that may be present. These patients are kept on the ventilator until their respiratory effort improves. This usually occurs as the patient's level of consciousness increases. Patients with more severe head injuries usually take longer to regain normal breathing efforts than patients with less severe injuries. The period of time it takes to regain the normal breathing pattern varies from patient to patient, taking anywhere from a few days to weeks.

Patients may be placed on the ventilator for other medical reasons as well. People with pre-existing lung disease or those who sustain lung damage at the time of the accident may require a ventilator until this damage resolves. Patients with pre-existing lung disease, such as emphysema, chronic bronchitis, or a history of extensive tobacco smoking, have the most difficult time; these patients are very difficult to get off the ventilator, because their lungs were already damaged before the accident. While such patients may have been getting by before the accident, they typically cannot tolerate any additional injury that affects the breathing effort. They are also at risk for additional damage, such as pneumonia, and as a result, are very dependent on the ventilator to breathe adequately. Several weeks may pass before they are able to breathe adequately without the assistance of the ventilator.

Patients on the ventilator are continually evaluated to assess both their need for the assistance provided by the ventilator and also their overall respiratory status. As a patient improves, the settings on the ventilator are slowly turned down. This is called **weaning the patient from the ventilator.** In effect, this is a process where the patient is encouraged to breathe more and more without help from the ventilator. This accomplishes two goals. First, by getting the patient to breathe without assistance from the ventilator, the patient gets stronger (like "weight lifting" for the lungs and breathing muscles). Second, by slowly withdrawing the ventilator's assistance, the patient's respiratory status can be systematically evaluated by the health care staff.

The **arterial blood gas** or **ABG** is used extensively during this process to check the amounts of oxygen and carbon dioxide in the arterial blood. The levels of these gases in the blood are good indicators of the respiratory "health" of the patient. Patients who are able to maintain normal oxygen levels in the blood without any additional oxygen usually have fairly healthy lungs. Likewise, normal carbon dioxide levels in patients who are not receiving extra breaths from the ventilator usually indicate that the ventilator can be removed. The breathing *rate* is also checked during the weaning process. Patients who appear to be working very hard to maintain normal breathing patterns must be weaned *slower* than those who appear to be breathing comfortably despite having the ventilator turned down. When patients show normal oxygen and carbon dioxide levels on the ABG, and appear to be breathing comfortably without the assistance of the ventilator, they are **extubated** (i.e., have the breathing tube removed) and taken off the ventilator.

Is it all right to talk to and touch the patient?

Yes. It would be an unusual situation for talking to or touching the patient to be harmful in any way. In fact, any additional stimuli, particularly the sound of a familiar voice or the feel of a gentle touch from a loved one, may help bring the patient out of unconsciousness. While this is not always the case, it certainly cannot hurt and is usually good for the family members in their attempt to deal with the tragedy at hand. Given the possible benefit for both the patient and the family, it probably should be encouraged. Care should be taken, however, not to dislodge any of the vital tubes or wires on or in the patient.

What does ischemia mean?

In general, **ischemia** describes a situation where cells are not getting enough oxygen and nutrients to survive. In the brain, the cells (**neurons**) are very sensitive to any amount of ischemia; this can occur if there is not enough blood (which carries the oxygen) reaching the brain from the heart, or when not enough oxygen is getting into the blood from the lungs. Anything that decreases the blood supply to the brain, such as a very low blood pressure from heart injury or severe infection, or high ICP (which acts to keep blood out of the brain), can cause ischemia. Severe pneumonia or lung injury can decrease the amount of oxygen that can get into the blood from the lungs, which can also lead to this problem.

Brain ischemia can also lead to further damage in the already injured patient, since neurons that do not receive enough oxygen begin to die after a period of time. If the ischemia is prolonged, it can result in a massive stroke. Once the neurons die, they do not regenerate and, if enough of them die, a significant loss of function could result, including death of the patient. Therefore, a large majority of the intensive treatment for head injury patients is concerned with identifying and correcting situations of ischemia before it can result in irreversible damage to areas in the brain that were not injured at the time of the accident. This treatment includes making sure there is enough oxygen in the blood and keeping the blood pressure high enough, as well as the ICP low enough, to maintain the necessary oxygen delivery to the brain.

What causes the patient to have a stroke?

The cells within the brain, called neurons, are very needy in that they require certain amounts of oxygen and nutrients. These cells quickly begin to die if they do not get enough nutrients, especially oxygen. The necessary oxygen is brought to the cells within the brain by the blood carried through the blood vessels. Oxygen is put into the blood in the lungs and then pumped through the blood vessels to the brain by the heart. The main artery to the brain, called the **internal carotid artery,** carries the oxygenated blood from the heart to the brain. Upon entering the brain, the internal carotid artery branches into smaller blood vessels that deliver the oxygen to the cells in the various lobes of the brain. A separate blood supply system, called the **vertebrobasilar system,** also helps to supply the brain with oxygen.

A stroke occurs when a portion of the brain does not receive enough oxygen. The neurons in the oxygen-starved area begin to die after about 4 to 7 minutes. Unless the needed oxygen supply is restored before that time, *irreversible* damage occurs to these cells. If enough neurons die, loss of function (such as the ability to move one side of the body, talk, or feel a certain part of the body) results. In general, the larger the number of dead neurons, the more significant the functional loss. Depending on the area involved, and the relative health of the surrounding, noninvolved area in terms of its oxygen supply, the patient may or may not recover some lost function.

Any situation leading to insufficient oxygen supply to the brain can result in a stroke. There are many different factors, all of which play a role in the oxygen delivery to the brain. As mentioned earlier, oxygen is carried by the blood. Therefore, there must be enough blood in the body to carry the necessary amounts of oxygen to the body and brain. Patients who suffer internal injuries or those who have significant bleeding as a result of the injury may not have enough blood to carry the oxygen. They may require a **blood transfusion** to receive the necessary amount of blood needed to meet the demands of the body and brain. In addition, the lungs must be functioning properly for the oxygen to get into the blood. Lung damage as a result of the injury or pneumonia, something very common in severe head injury patients, can impair the lung's ability to deliver oxygen to the blood. The use of the ventilator may be very useful in these situations to improve the oxygenation as the blood flows through the lungs.

Once the oxygen is put into the blood by the lungs, the heart must pump the oxygenated blood to the brain. Damage to the heart, which can occur in motor vehicle accidents when the patient's chest hits the steering wheel, or in older patients who have pre-existing heart conditions, can impair the heart's ability to produce enough pressure to get the blood into the brain. Cerebral edema (swelling within the brain) may significantly increase the pressure within the brain (the ICP). Even though the heart may be completely healthy, if the ICP is too high, the heart may have difficulty overcoming that pressure and fail to get enough blood into the brain. This is a major cause of strokes in head injury patients and is also thought to be a major contributor to the secondary damage (i.e., damage that occurs within the brain after the accident) in head injury patients.

Another possible cause of strokes results from damage to the blood vessels that carry the oxygen to the brain. Partial or complete tears in the blood vessels usually occur within the neck in the main artery to the brain (internal carotid artery). This injury, called an **internal carotid artery dissection,** can result in less blood getting to the brain. As the body tries to repair the "hole" in the artery, it forms a blood clot at the location of the injury. Small pieces of this blood clot can dislodge from the neck and travel in the blood going to the brain. These small blood clots, called **emboli,** may become stuck in the small arteries within the brain. This completely blocks the blood flow through the affected artery. The part of the brain receiving blood from that artery no longer receives the necessary oxygen and a stroke may result.

What are NG tubes and Dobhoff tubes? What do they do?

An NG tube is a naso (nose) gastric (stomach) tube; that is, a tube placed through the nose that goes down the back of the throat and **esophagus** until it reaches the stomach. Many patients with head injury have decreased levels of consciousness and frequently vomit. The patient is much too confused to vomit properly and is at risk for **aspirating** the **vomitus.** If this happens, the patient can develop severe pneumonia or **chemical pneumonitis.** To avoid this an NG tube is used. This allows the physician to empty out the stomach ("pump the stomach") so if the patient vomits there is nothing left to aspirate. An NG tube can be left in place for several days and can also be used to give medications. Many patients are unable to swallow pills, so the NG tube can be used to deliver the medicine into the stomach.

A Dobhoff tube is similar to an NG tube except it is smaller and passes through the stomach and into the small intestine. This tube does *not* empty out the stomach and is used as a delivery tube for medicines and food supplements. The Dobhoff tube does not prevent aspiration of vomitus—it is only a means of medicating and feeding the patient.

What is an arterial line?

This is similar to an intravenous line except it is placed in an artery rather than a vein. This line is not used for giving medication but rather to continuously monitor the patient's blood pressure. In order to effectively treat a patient with a severe head injury, it is essential to have an accurate measure of the blood pressure. An arterial line also gives the physician access to arterial blood, the blood coming from the heart and lungs. Since arterial blood is oxygenated, the physician can measure the oxygen and see tell how well the lungs and ventilator are working. Frequent arterial blood samples are taken and sent to the laboratory; the results of these tests guide the healthcare team in adjusting the ventilator and also help them decide when the patient can be extubated. Like all other lines and monitors, the arterial line may become clogged or dislodged and need to be replaced. Since these lines may become infected, patients are carefully monitored for any such signs. Many physicians will change the arterial line site after a few days to prevent this situation. Arterial line infection is rare but can cause serious problems, such as **sepsis.**

What is a central line?

A central line is essentially a large intravenous catheter placed in one of the large veins of the neck or chest that leads to the heart. A central line allows rapid delivery of fluid, blood, and medicine to the patient. It also can be used to monitor the patient's overall fluid status. This information can help avoid dehydration or overhydration. A central line is an important tool in the care of critically injured patients.

While helpful in treating patients, there are risks associated with the use of these lines. The veins in the neck and chest are very close to the lungs; occasionally, the lung can be accidentally punctured with the needle and this will cause a pneumothorax. A pneumothorax is essentially collapse of the lung. This problem can be corrected by insertion of a tube into the chest to re-expand the lung. Fortunately, this complication is rare. Another risk associated with central lines is infection of the line. For this reason, the central line is inserted under sterile conditions and a large sterile dressing covers the site at all times. The line is usually removed and a new line inserted every few days. These two methods help to prevent central line infections.

What is mannitol?

Mannitol is a drug that helps decrease swelling in the brain. It draws water out of the brain and into the bloodstream. The overall effect is to lower ICP. Mannitol helps to *prevent* secondary brain damage due to swelling that occurs after the injury, but it does not *repair* damage from the initial wound. The effectiveness of mannitol is limited and only works up to a certain point. In the period immediately after the injury, mannitol is very helpful in lowering the ICP, but is less effective as time passes.

What do Norcuron and morphine do?

Norcuron and morphine are medicines frequently used in head injury patients. Norcuron, also known as vecuronium, is a drug that causes *total* paralysis of all the muscles in the body. This effect lasts only a few hours so, to maintain paralysis, the drug must be given frequently or continuously through an intravenous line. Morphine is a drug that causes heavy sedation and pain relief. Norcuron should not be used without a sedative because doing so would leave the patient awake but unable to move. Imagine being awakened completely paralyzed and not being able to do anything about it! Now that we know what these drugs do, we must know when and why they are used in treating head injury. These drugs can be used to help control elevated ICP. Many head injury patients are wildly combative because they have difficulty processing external stimuli. This excitability can dramatically increase the patient's ICP. By sedating the patient, a mellowing effect is produced, which leads to lower pressures inside the head.

Another reason for using paralysis and sedation is to help in mechanical ventilation. Many patients have severe lung problems and cannot breathe on their own; they require a ventilator to do the breathing for them. Paralysis and sedation help to improve the efficiency of the breathing machine by allowing complete expansion of the lungs. A third reason to use morphine is that many of the patients have very painful injuries. Pain must be avoided for two reasons. First, patients should never suffer unnecessarily and morphine is an excellent way to relieve pain. Second, pain can lead to agitation and elevation in ICP. By alleviating pain, we get the secondary benefit of lowering the ICP.

How do you know how much Norcuron to give?

The patient's muscles must be adequately paralyzed, whether to facilitate the actions of the ventilator or to help decrease the ICP. Norcuron can be given at regularly scheduled intervals or continuously via an intraveneous catheter. It is given until the muscles are completely relaxed and unable to move. To check whether or not the medication is effectively doing its job a special device is used that stimulates muscles to contract (i.e., to move). The muscles twitch only slightly if the Norcuron is effective (normally, the muscles give a much stronger twitch). This muscle stimulator is also used to make sure that too much Norcuron is not given, since this can be harmful to the patient. Thus the information obtained from the muscle stimulator is used to adjust the amount of Norcuron given to the patient.

What is the difference between Norcuron and Pentobarbital?

Both medications may be used in the treatment of head injury. Although they have different effects within the body, both medications make the patient appear the same—they both induce chemical paralysis. Patients on these medications will be completely motionless even if their injuries have not damaged the motor system. **Norcuron** belongs to a group of drugs that inactivate all the muscles in the body, including the breathing muscles. Patients on Norcuron (and other similar chemical paralytics) must be on the ventilator or they will not be able to breathe. This medication is used in patients who have serious lung injuries in which it is important to let the ventilator do all the work of breathing until the lungs recover. It is also used in cases where it is difficult to control ICP. By chemically relaxing all the muscles in the body, Norcuron can sometimes be very helpful in decreasing elevated ICPs, thereby improving the blood supply to the injured brain.

Pentobarbital is a completely different medication, but it is also used in patients who have ICPs that are difficult to control. This medication is thought to protect the brain while it is injured, but just how this is done is unclear. Although the use of **pentobarbital coma** for head injury patients is controversial, in that it remains to be proven whether it truly leads to better recoveries, it is effective in decreasing out-of-control ICPs in some patients. This medication, in effect, puts the brain to sleep placing the patient in a very deep chemical coma. This can be thought of as somewhat similar to "suspended animation," in which the brain is protected until it recovers from the injury it sustained. Once the brain appears to be recovering, the pentobarbital is slowly reduced while the patient is watched carefully.

How do you know how much pentobarbital to give?

Pentobarbital is given to control the ICP until the brain recovers. Therefore, if the ICP is controlled, enough pentobarbital has been given. The same controversy that surrounds the use of pentobarbital also surrounds the question as to how much to give the patient. Some physicians use the EEG tracings to determine when enough pentobarbital has been given. The EEG measures the electrical activity within different parts of the brain (used to diagnose certain kinds of seizure disorders). A normal EEG recording has multiple spikes on all the line tracings obtained. As the pentobarbital begins to take effect, these line tracings become flattened, suggesting that the brain's electrical activity is decreased. Therefore, some physicians use this information to determine when the brain is chemically "asleep" or electrically inactive; others may continue to give pentobarbital to patients who have continued elevated ICP, despite an EEG recording that suggests that the brain is asleep. The additional pentobarbital is sometimes more effective in controlling the elevated ICP. As with any medication, care must be taken when this drug is administered to the patient. Blood pressure can drop very low if the dosage is too high or if it is given too quickly. Due to the potentially serious side effects of this medication, of which low blood pressure is one, it is usually only used as a last resort.

What does putting the patient into pentobarbital coma do? Does it wear off and, if so, how long does it take?

Pentobarbital is a very powerful drug that acts much the same as the combination of morphine and Norcuron. It has some extra effects on the brain not seen with Norcuron and morphine. Pentobarbital is thought to decrease the metabolic demands on the brain, essentially placing it in a state of suspended animation. Therefore, we say that the patient is in a pentobarbital coma. It is often very effective at lowering ICP. However, the use of pentobarbital requires a great deal of caution because there are many complications associated with its use, plus its ability to improve a patient's overall *outcome* has never been proven. For these reasons, pentobarbital is generally reserved for use as a last resort in those patients who do not respond to other treatments.

Patients placed in a pentobarbital coma require extremely close monitoring. Blood must be drawn one to two times per day to measure the amount of pentobarbital in the system. The level of pentobarbital must be carefully regulated to make sure the patient is receiving the correct dose. Each patient's metabolism is unique, so a certain dose for one person may be completely inadequate for another. One of the more common, and certainly the most devastating, complications associated with the use of pentobarbital is **hypotension.**

Hypotension is caused by the relaxing effect the drug has on the heart and the body's blood vessels. The drop in blood pressure can be extremely rapid and very severe. This can be damaging to the brain because, when the blood pressure drops, less blood reaches the brain. When less blood reaches the brain, the neurons are deprived of the oxygen they need to survive. For this reason, all patients about to be placed into pentobarbital coma must be in an ICU and the drug must be given very slowly. Monitoring devices, such as Swan-Ganz catheters, arterial lines, and ICP monitors, are all essential in safely administering this drug. Patients may also be monitored with EEG recordings to check brain wave activity. The EEG recording can help decide if the patient is receiving enough pentobarbital. In general, a sufficient dose must be given to control the ICP until the brain begins to recover.

Another problem associated with using pentobarbital is infection. All patients in the ICU are susceptible to infections, but pentobarbital coma patients are at much higher risk. Some feel that the drug actually causes a blunting of a person's immune response, so if an infection develops, the patient's ability to fight that infection is much lower than normal. Further, the drug depresses the signs of infection. Most people develop a fever when they have an infection; pentobarbital essentially turns off the mechanism in the brain that controls body temperature. Hence, a patient in a pentobarbital coma can have a raging infection, yet exhibit a normal or even low body temperature. Pentobarbital can completely disrupt the brain's thermostat mechanism and the body temperature can drop significantly. These patients often require special heating blankets to maintain normal body temperature. Skin breakdown is another problem because the patient may lie in bed without moving for days; pressure sores can result if the patient is not routinely turned and carefully padded.

Eventually, it will be time to take the person out of the coma. The drug wears off slowly over a period of hours to days. Since there is much variation in the body's ability to clear the drug, the time period will be different for each patient. Generally, the drug level drops approximately 5 to 10 points per day. Hence, the time it takes for the drug's effect to resolve can be estimated by knowing the pentobarbital level at the time the infusion was stopped. Drug levels are closely monitored even after the drug infusion is stopped. This is to determine when the patient is no longer under the effects of the drug. When the level of drug is low enough (usually below 10), a neurologic assessment of the patient can be done. Examinations performed before the drug level is sufficiently low are considered invalid because the patient is still artificially sedated due to the effects of the pentobarbital. Until the neurologic examination is accurate (i.e., the pentobarbital level is at least below 10), there is really no way to predict the patient's prognosis.

Why are you checking the pupils and pinching the patient regularly?

Patients, especially those with more severe head injuries, are often unconscious. Therefore, methods other than asking questions must be employed to evaluate the patient's condition. Although unconscious, certain automatic responses still function and enable some insight as to the function and overall health of the brain. These automatic responses, called **reflexes,** include the pupil's response to light. Normally, the pupils get smaller in bright light. Damage to one of the nerves, called the oculomotor nerve, that go to the eye prevents this normal response to light; the pupil remains large and does not respond to light in these cases. This is very important because this nerve (i.e., the **oculomotor nerve,** which causes the pupil to get smaller with light) is adjacent to the brain stem. Located within the brain stem is the life control center, which is absolutely necessary for sustaining life. Compression of this nerve by an abnormally swollen brain causes it to malfunction. Therefore, this can be used as an early sign that the brain is beginning to press up against the life control center (called herniation), a situation that, left untreated, can quickly damage this center and lead to death.

Just as the pupil's response to light is a valuable method for checking the patient's condition, so is the patient's response to painful stimuli. Due to the unconscious state of many head injury patients, some noxious stimuli must be given to get the patient to respond. Pinching the patient is the usual method to elicit a response. While other less painful methods could be used, patients who are deeply unconscious will not likely respond to these stimuli. It is important to get the patient's "best" response to accurately assess the health and function of the brain. Unfortunately, a painful stimulus is often necessary to get these patients to respond. Certain responses suggest better function than others. For example, patients who move to remove the examiner's pinching fingers (i.e., purposeful) are generally doing better than those who display more automatic movements (such as extending the arms and legs to painful stimuli). These responses are used to assess the condition of the patient. Those that appear to be demonstrating movements considered to be worse than those shown before are given more treatment and further investigation is held to determine the cause of the decline.

Patients can continue to have injury occurring within the brain after the initial accident. The initial injury usually causes the brain to swell and may have caused bleeding within the brain. This means that the injury process within the brain continues for days after the initial injury. The length of time in which this secondary damage process occurs is dependent on the severity of the initial injury and the overall condition of the patient at any given time. The goal of therapy is to prevent as much further damage as possible in an attempt to preserve as much function as possible. One very valuable method for watching these patients is with serial neurologic examinations. These examinations, which include checking the pupils and testing the patient's response to pain, help to give insight as to the condition and function of the brain. The general trend of the patient's responses enables the health care medical staff to determine if the patient is getting better or worse.

Due to the fact that the injury process can continue to evolve after the initial accident, it is important to observe these patients very closely. A change in the pupil response to light or the patient's response to painful stimuli can help alert the health care staff that something is changing. This may, in turn, prompt another CT scan or new treatments in an effort to protect the healthy parts of the brain and preserve as much function as possible. The CT scan may identify a new area of bleeding or compression that can be treated successfully with an emergency operation.

How long will the patient be in the ICU and where does the patient go from there?

The ICU is where severely injured patients, or those who the health care staff want to watch more closely, are admitted when they are brought to the hospital. It is where the most aggressive and intense management of head injury patients occurs. Most ICUs are equipped to handle just about anything, including some surgical procedures, and to handle whatever else may happen in the course of therapy. In most ICUs, one nurse is responsible for only one patient, which allows for more one-on-one care. Patients remain in the ICU as long as they require intensive medical treatment or are in a situation where they must be observed very closely. This includes patients with significant cerebral edema, those who require the breathing machine, patients who have an ICP monitor or ventriculostomy, those with major infections, or those who have multiple large contusions (bruises) within the brain. In the absence of major infection, multiple internal organ dysfunction, and lung problems, the average length of stay in the ICU for a severe head injury patient ranges from 10 to 21 days. Patients with less severe head injuries spend less time in the ICU, while those with compounding factors, such as multiple organ dysfunction or lung problems requiring the assistance of the breathing machine (ventilator), often are in the ICU for a longer period of time.

When patients have been stabilized and no longer require intensive management, they are transferred out of the ICU. Those with severe head injury who remain in an unconscious state may be transferred to a **step-down unit.** Patients are transferred to this unit when they are not sick enough to be in an ICU but who still require more supervised care than can be provided on a typical hospital floor. Typically, there are more than two patients in a room, with one nurse taking care of two or more patients at a time. Patients with less severe injuries or those who do not need as much supervised care are transferred from the ICU (or from the step-down unit when they are ready) to a regular hospital room (also called the "floor"). Usually there are two patients per room and the patients have more autonomy than in the ICU or step-down unit setting.

Donna: Sharon was in intensive care for about 3 weeks. Then she went to what they called a step-down unit. She was still in a coma and wasn't responding to anything, although her arms moved up and down uncontrollably. And she had this horrible lung infection, cytomegalovirus. Oh, God, that was terrible. They had done a tracheotomy while she was in the ICU, and now they had to stick this tube down there and clean out the phlegm. The nurses always advised us to step out of the room when they were clearing her lungs.

One time I said, "Oh, I think I can handle this," but I started gagging! It really is best to leave the room for many of the routine tests and tasks. I think it just makes you sadder to see that kind of thing, because it drives home the point that the patient is out of control . . . to have other people doing every bodily function for her that normally her body took care of on its own. To watch that just increased my sadness. And in that particular instant, the reality was that the smell just about made me throw up. I recommend that everyone be aware of what the health care professionals are going to do; ask questions. Ask everything you can think of, "What are you going to do? How's her temperature? How's her infection? What kind of antibiotics is she on? Why is she on so many?" Learn as much as you can about what they're doing. But when they're wanting to clean up the patient or change tubes or whatever, get out. It may not be a good thing for you to see.

CHAPTER
8

Other Medical Issues

One important aspect of taking care of a patient who has sustained a head injury is caring for the *entire* patient. Each patient has his or her specific medical history, such as heart problems, diabetes, or drug and alcohol abuse problems. A person with a head injury has altered consciousness and is usually unable to tell health care staff about his or her medical past. All this information is vitally important since it affects the treatments that health care staff can use. Because the patient is unable to report this information to the health care staff, it becomes the responsibility of the family members to try and provide as much information as possible about the patient's medical history.

Some easy ways to do this are to (1) make a list of the patient's doctors and give it to the medical team, (2) report any drug or alcohol problems (this information will be kept confidential), and (3) bring the patient's home medications to the hospital and give them to the nurse. **Do not give the medicine to the patient.**

There are many problems associated with head injury. Most head injuries result from violent collisions, such as motor vehicle accidents, falls, and assaults. These types of accidents are directed against the entire body so frequently the patient has *multiple* injuries that need special attention. It is very common for head injury patients to have broken bones or injuries to the organs inside the abdomen or chest. At times these injuries can be more of a threat to the patient's life than the head injury. Injuries to the heart or lungs and internal abdominal bleeding must be fixed quickly to prevent shock and death. These wounds make recovery longer and more difficult.

Patients with **isolated head injuries** commonly have injuries to bones of the face and the **cervical spine.** These injuries require immediate attention as they can be potentially life threatening. Severe fractures to the bones of the face may block a patient's airway and not allow proper breathing. Cervical spine fractures are a threat to the spinal cord, which, when damaged, can leave a person permanently paralyzed. When a patient with a serious head injury is found, the first thing the **Emergency Medical Service** team does is stabilize the patient's neck with a hard collar and insert a tube in the patient's throat to prevent blockage of the airway. The patient is then brought to a hospital for further stabilization and care of the multiple injuries.

Once the patient is examined in the emergency department, he or she is sent to the **intensive care unit** or **ICU** or sometimes directly to the operating room. The ICU is well suited to the specific needs of these critically injured patients. There are a variety of machines that monitor the patients, breathe for the patients, and administer vital medicines. However, despite these lifesaving machines, there are many problems associated with being in an ICU for a long period of time. Infection is a constant threat, but especially worrisome for patients with head injuries. **Pneumonia, urinary tract infections,** and **sepsis** are very common in patients who are bed-bound in the ICU. Many head injury patients **aspirate** at the scene of an accident, and this predisposes them for developing pneumonia.

The monitors, drains, and tubes needed to care for the patients in the ICU all bypass many of the natural defenses that ward off infection. Intravenous lines puncture the skin, Foley catheters are placed in the bladder, and breathing tubes provide a direct portal of entry to the lungs. Bacteria can grow in these foreign devices and gain entry into the blood (sepsis), bladder (urinary tract infections), and lungs (pneumonia). Antibiotics can be used but are not always effective against the hearty bacteria that live in the ICU. The best defense against infection is prevention and that is why these lines and tubes must be changed frequently. Nurses and respiratory therapists are constantly suctioning out and putting special medicines into the breathing tube to keep the airway clean. Despite these aggressive measures, anyone who is bedridden in the ICU will likely get some type of infection. For this reason, routine tests are done when the patient develops a fever or shows other signs of infection. Blood, urine, and **sputum** are sent to the hospital's laboratory to determine if there is infection. The lab will be able to identify the infection and recommend an appropriate antibiotic, specifically designed to kill the infecting bacteria. Usually, we win the battle, but infections can cause serious delays in a patient's recovery and can even be fatal, particularly in the elderly. One of the easiest and most effective ways to decrease infection in the ICU is to wash your hands upon entering and leaving the patient's room. Hand washing has been proven to be one of the most effective ways to prevent infection.

The brain can be thought of as the body's computer center; it oversees almost every bodily function. The heart, kidneys, lungs, and bowels are all directly and indirectly under the control of the brain. Because of this intimate relationship with other parts of the body, patients with brain injuries are at risk of developing problems with these other systems. One common problem seen in brain injured patients is **disseminated intravascular coagulation** or **DIC,** which is when the body's system that controls blood clotting is damaged. The blood loses the ability to clot properly and abnormal bleeding and/or clotting can be present. This is a very serious problem since it can increase bleeding inside the brain, furthering the damage. There is no completely effective treatment. The presence of DIC is associated with some of the more severe forms of brain injury.

Another common problem in patients with head injury is abnormalities in the blood's **electrolyte** content. The electrolytes are chemical elements in the blood used by the cells of the body for energy. They are usually found in specific quantities closely regulated by the brain. When injured, the brain loses its ability to properly monitor and correct the concentrations of these electrolytes and the entire system breaks down. The blood is the transport system in the body. Think of it as a system of delivery trucks traveling across the country. When the normal electrolyte concentrations are disrupted, the entire transport system is affected. The trucks have the wrong cargo and don't know where to go. This can result in problems with any and all organs in the body.

A further complication of head injury is the development of seizures. These can occur right after the head injury or can appear up to 2 months later. Seizures are very dramatic and often are described by observers as being scary to watch. They can range from a simple rhythmic twitching of the face or hand to a violent shaking of the entire body. **Posttraumatic seizures** are common in 35% of severe head injuries. Patients are often given a medicine called **phenytoin** or **Dilantin** to protect against seizures. This medication is generally very effective in controlling seizures, although some patients still have seizures despite taking this medicine. Trauma to the brain causes a change in the normal structure of the cells of the brain. The brain was previously described as the body's central computer; a seizure is essentially a short circuit in the computer. Seizures must be controlled because they put a severe stress on a brain that has already been injured. If left untreated, seizures can lead to further brain injury. A single seizure immediately after a blow to the head is fairly common, and drug treatment is usually not started unless the patient's computed tomography or CT scan shows brain injury or the patient has further seizures.

Most serious brain injury patients spend a long time in the ICU and are bedridden as a result of their injuries. The body was not designed to lie in bed for long periods of time and many of the procedures in the ICU are done to prevent the problems associated with prolonged bed rest. The practice of suctioning the **endotracheal tube** was described in Chapter 7. Normally, the body has defenses to keep the body's airway clear, such as coughing, sneezing, and swallowing. A person with a brain injury loses the ability to perform these basic cleansing mechanisms and soon the airway becomes clogged with mucus and debris. Suctioning allows the nurse to clean the airway and prevent infection and blockage of the airway.

Lying in bed also causes the blood to flow more slowly through the body, particularly in the legs. Normal activities, such as walking, stretching, and bending, help pump blood through our legs and back to the heart. This keeps the blood moving and prevents it from pooling or slowing down. The body can do this job of pumping while we sleep or sit at a desk for long periods but, eventually, the blood begins to pool. When the blood slows down and pools, it increases the chance of the blood clotting. People who are confined to bed are at increased risk of having their blood form clots, especially in their legs. The term for these blood clots is **deep vein thromboses** or **DVTs.** These clots are dangerous because pieces of clot can break off and travel through the bloodstream into the lungs and cause **pulmonary embolism.** This, in turn, may result in serious breathing problems, or even fatal lung damage.

Blood thinners can be given to break up the clots, but often these cannot be used safely in people with head injury because they may increase the chances of the patient bleeding *inside* the brain. A second option is to surgically insert a filter into the main blood vessel coming from the legs to catch the blood clots. The best option is prevention and that is why every head injury patient is given **subcutaneous heparin,** wears **pneumatic air stockings,** and undergoes physical therapy while in bed. The heparin thins the blood enough to decrease the chance of developing a DVT without increasing the risk of bleeding in the brain and the pneumatic air stockings and physical therapy help to pump the blood and prevent it from pooling.

One final issue that comes up with serious brain injury patients is the need for feeding tubes and more permanent breathing tubes called **tracheostomies.** Many of these patients require long-term breathing support and are unable to swallow. The endotracheal tube provides a very good airway but it cannot be left in place for long periods of time. The endotracheal tube enters the mouth or nose and passes down through the **larynx** (voice box) into the **trachea** (windpipe). After about 2 weeks, scarring may develop in the larynx. To avoid this, patients often must have a tracheostomy inserted. This is a surgical procedure in which a small, more permanent tube is put directly into the trachea below the larynx. This allows the same respiratory care without the potential damage to the voice mechanism.

The purpose of all the previously mentioned treatments is to help the patient recover from injury. Nutrition plays a key role because the body cannot heal itself without food. The dietary needs of head injury patients are extremely important, since many require *more than double their normal dietary intake*. For this reason, they are fed through a small tube inserted through the nose and into the stomach. This tube also allows nurses to give medications that cannot be given through the intravenous lines. While these tubes work well for the first week or two, there are some problems associated with their use. They are very small and frequently clog, especially with thicker medicines. They can also irritate the skin in the nose and cause ulcers and skin breakdown. A solution to these problems is a feeding tube placed directly into the stomach through the abdominal wall. This procedure is done by a general surgeon or gastroenterologist in a specialized operating room. The feeding tube is larger and is less inclined to clog. With this tube, the patient can begin to eat by mouth in addition to receiving tube feedings. Thus the patient can slowly relearn how to chew and swallow without missing any meals. Both the tracheostomy and feeding tube can be removed when the patient no longer needs them.

❧ COMMONLY ASKED QUESTIONS ❧

What medications will be needed long term?

Various medications are used in the treatment of head injury patients. Most of these are only necessary during the more acute stages while the patient is in the hospital. For instance, **mannitol,** a medication given to help decrease the brain swelling and subsequent elevated **intracranial pressures** or **ICPs,** is only used when the brain is still swollen. As the swelling and the ICPs begin to decrease, mannitol is no longer necessary. The same is true for the intravenous fluid the patient typically receives. As the patient begins to recover, or if a feeding tube has been placed, intravenous fluids are no longer necessary.

There are other medications, however, that might have to be administered for a certain time period even after leaving the hospital. This is dependent on the particular circumstances surrounding the patient's condition. Head injury patients are typically put on medications called **anticonvulsants** that help to prevent seizures. Dilantin is one commonly used anticonvulsant. Patients with head injury are at risk of having a seizure. Although there is some controversy about this, most patients are placed on an antiseizure medication, such as Dilantin, for 10 to 14 days after the accident even though there may have been no evidence of seizure activity. This is a situation where an ounce of prevention is worth a pound of cure. The patients are taken off the medication after the 10 to 14 day period if no seizures occur.

Despite the antiseizure medication, some patients continue to have seizures while others may develop a problem with seizures a relatively long period after the injury. These are thought to occur secondary to the scar that forms when the brain attempts to repair the damaged area. This area becomes a short circuit of sorts and can lead to seizure activity. Patients who develop seizures long after the accident are typically placed on anticonvulsants if they persist and may require these antiseizure medications for life. In addition, people who have more than one seizure while in the hospital may be kept on anticonvulsants for up to 6 months after the injury. If the patient shows no evidence of seizure activity after this period of time, the medication is slowly reduced while the patient is watched for any seizure activity.

Additional medications may be necessary for periods longer than the hospitalization. Medications used to help the food move through the intestines may be necessary for longer periods of time, especially in patients who are not walking around; the same is true for stool softeners and other medications that help patients have bowel movements.

Some patients develop high blood pressure after head injury, and medication may be necessary to keep this under control. This is particularly important for patients who have a blood clot within the brain tissue. Although **antihypertensives** may initially be necessary to help prevent enlargement of these blood clots (by keeping the blood pressure under control), such medications are usually not necessary for very long periods after leaving the hospital. This is not true, however, for patients who had blood pressure problems prior to the accident. In general, any medication that was necessary before the accident will still be necessary after the accident.

Why does the patient need to be given blood?

Patients who have suffered severe traumatic injuries are often very sick. Many have multiple injuries and are highly unstable. The physician's job is to provide the injured body with everything it needs to heal itself. Many times the body is unable to support itself and the health care team has to take over for the nonfunctioning systems of the body. For example, the ventilator takes over for the lungs when they are unable to provide enough oxygen for the patient.

Blood is vital for life. Many trauma patients lose blood at the time of their injury through internal or external bleeding. The body does not have an unlimited supply of blood. The entire body contains about 5 liters of blood (about 2½ gallons). Many times the patient's **hematocrit** level will be too low, indicating the loss of blood. If it gets too low, it may interfere with oxygen delivery to the brain and other organs. None of the cells in the body can live without oxygen for very long, so giving the patient blood helps to keep the hematocrit at a normal level. This, in turn, ensures that all the cells of the body get the oxygen they need to survive.

Why do you need to change sites of intravenous lines, Camino monitors, and ventriculostomies?

Seriously head-injured patients require careful monitoring. Many of the treatments and medications used to help these patients change from moment to moment. The monitors, intravenous lines, and drains are all vital instruments to ensure proper medical and surgical management. Unfortunately, in order to gain accurate information about what is happening inside the head or body, we need to place indwelling devices. Indwelling refers to a medical device (monitor, catheter, or probe) that lies partly inside and partly outside the body. This creates a kind of double-edged sword. The information gained from indwelling devices is much more accurate than probes completely outside the body. However, any time a device is placed through the protective barrier of the skin, the patient is at risk of developing an infection. Bacteria that live on the skin can travel along the outside of the catheter and work their way into the body. This can happen with central lines, intravenous lines, Foley catheters, Camino monitors, ventriculostomies, and virtually *any* device that has been passed through the skin. The longer these devices are left in place, the higher the chance for infection. For this reason, the physician attempts to remove these devices as soon as possible. If they are required for medical decision making for more than a few days, the device should be changed and the site of insertion moved whenever possible. Changing these monitors and lines helps control the rate of infection.

What is Dilantin?

Dilantin or phenytoin is a drug that helps control seizures. The medicine works directly on the cell of the brain to block seizure activity. Seizures are frequently caused by head injuries, so patients with a serious head injury need to be placed on Dilantin for a certain period of time. Some patients are put on Dilantin even though they never have had a seizure. This is a precaution for anyone suspected of having a brain injury. If the patient remains seizure-free, he or she can be slowly taken off the drug. Not everyone who is hit in the head needs Dilantin; it is generally reserved for those patients with more severe injuries.

Is it common to have seizures after a head injury? Do they eventually go away?

Seizures are seen in about 35% of all serious brain injuries. Seizures that occur after head trauma are the result of damage to focal areas of the brain. The injured area undergoes changes that result in an area of increased excitability. This area becomes independent from the rest of the brain and begins to send out signals on its own. These signals can be picked up by the rest of the brain and result in a short circuit of the entire nervous system. The result is a massive outpouring of independent synchronized neurologic signals that produce violent shaking, strange eye movements, and a variety of other abnormal sensations. Seizures are dangerous because they put an enormous stress on an already injured brain. Controlling these violent convulsions is extremely important. There are a variety of medications designed to control seizures. It is not uncommon for patients to be given anticonvulsants prophylactically to prevent seizures from developing.

Seizures occurring after a brain injury (posttraumatic epilepsy) are classified into three types. There is immediate, early, and late epilepsy. Immediate epilepsy refers to convulsive behaviors that occur at the time of, or within minutes of, the initial brain trauma. These tend not to recur and often require no therapy whatsoever. The prognosis is good and most patients will never have another seizure. Early epilepsy refers to the development of seizures within the first week after a brain injury. This type of epilepsy tends to result from more serious head injuries in which there has been visible structural damage to the brain (contusions, hemorrhages, depressed fractures, or in-driven foreign bodies). About one fourth of the adult patients with early seizures go on to develop long-term epilepsy. The percentage is somewhat higher in children. Most of these patients will be on anticonvulsant medication for the rest of their lives. Late epilepsy refers to seizures that occur anytime after the first week and sometimes don't happen until years after the initial injury. The long-term outcome of these patients is similar to those in the early epilepsy group.

What does a seizure look like?

There are many different types of seizures that can result after a head injury. The most common form of posttraumatic seizure, as well as the most dramatic, is the tonic-clonic (grand mal) seizure. This seizure is characterized by the patient's body going stiff, with loss of consciousness, incontinence, clenching of the teeth, and then violent shaking of the entire body that lasts 10 to 15 seconds or longer. After the seizure, the patient is confused, sleepy, and glassy eyed. This period after the seizure, also known as the postictal phase, may last for minutes to hours.

There are other seizures that are much more discrete and sometimes may even evade detection. Patients may simply "zone out" for a few seconds and then abruptly regain consciousness. Other seizures present themselves as rhythmic beating of an arm or leg without any change in the patient's level of consciousness. Even though they are not as dramatic as grand mal seizures they still signify abnormal brain discharges and should be controlled with medication.

How are the patient's lungs?

This question is very common because many head injury patients have respiratory problems. Many times these problems are a result of direct trauma, such as a punctured lung. Other times they come from infection, such as pneumonia, which results from **aspiration** caused by the patient's diminished level of consciousness. The lungs take time to heal but, more often than not, they get better. Chest x-ray films are frequently taken to monitor the lungs for pneumonias, **pneumothoraces,** and other signs of lung problems. Arterial blood samples are taken to make sure proper gas exchange is occurring in the lungs. Remember that the breathing machine can move air in and out of the lungs, but oxygen must still move into the bloodstream through normal physiologic mechanisms in the lung tissue.

Why does the patient get pneumonia? How can you tell if
it is getting better?

Pneumonia is common in any intensive care patient. The incidence may be even higher in head injury patients who often aspirate at the time of the injury. The fluid aspirated into the lungs can lead to an **aspiration pneumonia,** which can decrease the lung's ability to function properly. Serial arterial blood gases or ABGs, which measure the amount of oxygen and carbon dioxide in the blood, are used to ascertain how well the lungs are working in the presence of the pneumonia. In addition to affecting lung function, serious pneumonias can lead to infections in other parts of the body as the blood flows through the infected lung and subsequently spreads the infection to additional locations.

The health care staff uses different signs to diagnose pneumonia. Patients with pneumonia may develop a large amount of thick, yellow-brown secretions within the lung. These secretions are detected when the endotracheal tube is suctioned in patients who are intubated. The development of high fevers (i.e., a temperature of 102° F or higher) is also indicative of some type of infection. The combination of high fevers and thick endotracheal secretions suggests that a pneumonia may be present. Chest x-rays films are also utilized to take a look at the lungs themselves. These images can identify areas suspicious for pneumonia. When the suspicion is high that a pneumonia is present, samples of the endotracheal secretions are sent to the laboratory for cultures. The presence of bacterial growth on the cultures is suggestive of a pneumonia or bronchial infection (infection in the breathing tubes rather than the lung tissue itself). Patients are then placed on antibiotics to treat the presumed pneumonia. The antibiotics chosen depend on the type of bacteria grown on the culture.

The same factors used to diagnose pneumonia, namely, the presence of thick secretions, fever, bacterial growth on culture, and chest x-ray film appearance, are also used to follow the pneumonia's course once antibiotic therapy is begun. As the pneumonia begins to improve, the fevers usually subside. The amount and thickness of the endotracheal secretions also decrease in time. The color of the secretions also typically returns to a more normal whitish color as the antibiotics begin to kill the bacteria responsible for the pneumonia. Repeat sputum (the secretion obtained from the endotracheal tube or the back of the throat) cultures also show no bacterial growth once the pneumonia is cleared up with the antibiotics. The chest x-ray film, which is the least sensitive test in following pneumonia, is the last to return to normal once the pneumonia has been treated. Patients who do not show improvement on the antibiotics may have developed another lung infection from a different type of bacteria that is not sensitive to the antibiotics originally selected. These patients may have persistent fevers and thick endotracheal secretions. Repeat cultures are obtained to identify the problem and new antibiotics are started as necessary.

What is a culture and what do you do with the results?

A culture is a laboratory test used to determine whether or not an infection is present. Samples of bodily fluids, such as blood, urine, oral secretions, and **cerebrospinal fluid** or **CSF,** are sent to the lab to see if there are any bacteria present within the sample. Normally, these fluids do not have any bacteria within them and thus the presence of any bacteria in these fluids is suggestive of an infection. In order to determine if there are bacteria present, small portions of the fluid sample are placed on special culture dishes. These dishes are filled with nutrients that bacteria need to grow. Bacterial growth on these cultures indicates that there are bacteria within the fluid sample and therefore suggests an infection is present. Not only do these cultures help diagnose an infection, they also identify the type of bacteria responsible for that infection. The health care staff then uses this information to select the most appropriate antibiotic for the patient. Repeat cultures can be used to follow the infection's response to the antibiotics selected. The absence of any bacterial growth on subsequent cultures indicates that the antibiotics being given to the patient are working.

How do you know what antibiotics to use?

Antibiotics are a group of different medicines that help to eliminate bacteria in treating infections. There are a wide range of antibiotics available, each of which is particularly good at killing various types of bacteria. Therefore, for the health care staff to select the appropriate antibiotic to give to the patient the bacteria responsible for the infection must first be identified. This is done through the use of cultures. Various fluids from the body are sent to the laboratory for culture. The bacteria that grow on these cultures are typically the ones responsible for the infection in the patient. The bacteria that grew are then tested with different antibiotics to determine which antibiotic the bacteria are most sensitive to (i.e., which antibiotic kills the particular type of bacteria the best). If the patient's infection does not respond to the initial antibiotic selected, additional antibiotics may be added or completely different antibiotics may be started. The patient is then monitored to assess the response to the treatment.

Why is the patient having breathing problems?

Many people with head injury are unconscious for a period of time after the accident. During this time they are often so deeply "asleep" that normal breathing does not occur. The patient may be able to take a few breaths, but not enough to supply the body with the necessary oxygen or deep enough to get rid of carbon dioxide waste. In addition to not breathing deeply or rapidly enough, patients who are deeply unconscious typically do not protect their airway. Oral secretions are thus able to get down into the lungs and cause aspiration pneumonia. In fact, it is very common for head injury patients to aspirate at the scene of the accident. The oral secretions that end up in the lungs can cause damage and lead to lung dysfunction; the resulting pneumonia can also be very difficult to treat.

The end result of either not breathing well enough or having lung damage from aspiration is **hypoxia** (not having enough oxygen in the blood and tissues of the body). The injured brain is very sensitive to any decreased amount of oxygen within the blood, which can quickly cause further damage in the brain. Therefore, it is extremely important to provide enough oxygen to the patient. The use of a ventilator helps to ensure that this is the case in those patients who are too sleepy to breathe adequately on their own. In addition, using the ventilator enables the health care staff to control the work of breathing. Fast breathing may be necessary on command to counteract elevated ICP (called hyperventilation), or deeper breaths may be necessary to help keep the lungs fully inflated. Therefore, the ventilator in a sense can play a role in the patient's therapy and treatment.

As patients begin to awaken from unconsciousness, they often breathe much more efficiently. When this occurs, the ventilator is adjusted so that the patients do all the work of breathing. Even though still on the ventilator, patients actually breathe without assistance. Those who appear to be able to breathe enough on their own have the ventilator and breathing tube removed. A small group of head injury patients, especially those with concurrent high cervical spinal cord injury, damage the actual breathing center in the brain stem and spinal cord. Irreversible damage to this area can result in permanent inability to breathe. If these patients survive the accident, which is typically not the case, they require a ventilator for the rest of their life. Again, this is the exception, not the rule, with head injury patients.

What about nutrition? How will you feed the patient?

Adequate nutrition is important, particularly in head injury patients. The metabolism increases significantly in these patients. As the metabolism increases, their nutritional requirements also increase. To keep up with these needs and to optimize the recovery process, adequate nutrition must be provided to these patients.

Head injury patients, however, are unable to provide themselves with this necessary nutrition. Unconscious patients obviously cannot eat by themselves. Those who are more alert but are intubated also have a very difficult time eating. The same is true for patients who may have sustained injuries to the mouth and/or face. Significant swelling or fractures involving the jaw can make it difficult to eat and swallow sufficient food to maintain necessary levels of nutrition. In these situations, in which the patient is either too lethargic to eat or is physically unable to get the food through the mouth into the stomach, nutritional assistance must be provided.

Nutrients can be administered in an intravenous form (i.e., given through an IV line). This is known as total parenteral nutrition or TPN. Despite its name, this method of nutritional supplementation is limited in the amount of nutrients that can be provided to the patient. Further, those receiving TPN have a higher incidence of infection compared to other methods of nutritional assistance. In some instances, however, this may be the only method available and, as such, has value in some cases.

It is generally agreed that the optimal route to deliver nutrition to these patients is into the stomach. This method follows the more "natural pathway" and, as such, has few or no side effects. The higher incidence of infection seen in patients who are receiving TPN is not seen in those receiving nutrition via this route. This method can be accomplished in several different ways. A tube can be passed through the mouth or nose and down into the stomach; the small flexible Dobhoff tube is most often used for this purpose. **Nasogastric** or **NG tubes** can also be used to get this nutrition into the stomach, but they have the disadvantage of being too rigid. This can result in tissue breakdown around the mouth or nose if the NG tube is left in place too long. Liquid nutrition, high in the necessary nutrients, is administered through these tubes directly into the stomach, where it begins to be absorbed by the body. There are various forms of this liquid nutrition, each with a different composition designed to address special needs of the patient.

In patients who continue to require nutritional assistance for longer periods of time, a feeding tube can be surgically placed into the stomach. This is called a **percutaneous endoscopic gastrostomy** or **PEG,** which is a tube with one end located in the stomach and the other on the surface of the abdomen. This long name describes the surgical method in which the feeding tube is placed. Percutaneous means through the skin, endoscopic refers to the fiberoptic telescope placed in the stomach, and gastrostomy is simply a hole in the stomach. The liquid nutrition can be administered through this surgically implanted tube, while bypassing the need to have any tubes in the mouth or nose. Much like a tracheostomy, a surgical procedure that often accompanies the placement of these feeding tubes, the PEG is not permanent. As the patients improve and begin to be able to provide themselves with sufficient nutrition, the PEG can be removed.

Is the patient getting enough nutrition?

The head injury patient and multiple injury patient both have increased caloric needs. These patients are often unable to eat so it is the physician's job to ensure that the patient gets enough nutrition. The use of Dobhoff and PEG feeding tubes are one way to ensure proper caloric intake. Another easy way is to weigh the patient on a daily basis to make sure he or she is not losing weight. All the medicines, intravenous fluids, and feedings given to a patient are recorded on a daily flow sheet by the nurses. This enables the physician to know exactly what the patient is receiving. The nutritional supplements administered through the feeding tube are specially formulated to meet the dietary needs of the injured patient; these supplements are high in calories and vitamins. There are many kinds and each one has a slightly different composition so a specific brand of supplement can be chosen to meet the specific needs of the patient.

Why does the patient need a "trach" and PEG? Are they permanent?

Tracheostomies and feeding tubes (or PEGs) are frequently used to take care of patients who have significant injuries requiring an extended convalescent period. Tracheostomies are small breathing tubes surgically placed in the trachea. They are placed below the level of the vocal cords. This protects the vocal cords from damage that would occur from an endotracheal tube left in place for more than 2 weeks. Having a tracheostomy does not mean that a patient has to be attached to a ventilator. Many patients with a tracheostomy need them for airway protection and not for help in breathing. Although tracheostomies are placed surgically, they are not always permanent. They can remain in place as long as the patient's condition warrants their use. As the patient begins to recover, a special attachment can be put on the tracheostomy that enables the patient to speak. Patients who recover and no longer require the assistance of a tracheostomy can have it removed. This is done in a slow step-by-step manner referred to as "downsizing the trach." After the tracheostomy is removed, the hole closes on its own in a few days. Therefore, the length of time a tracheostomy remains in place is very much dependent on the patient's condition.

Feeding tubes are placed to ensure that the patient gets enough nutrition throughout the recovery period. It is very important for the patient to receive enough vitamins and nutrients to help heal the wounds. Many patients with head injuries are unable to eat for long periods of time because of their altered level of consciousness. These patients would starve and never recover without proper nutrition. Dobhoff tubes can be placed through the mouth or nose and advanced down the esophagus into the stomach. These tubes are a good temporary measure but they frequently get clogged and displaced. Patients who require longer term tube feedings are better served with a PEG tube. A PEG tube is larger than the Dobhoff tube and is less likely to clog. It is also easily removed when the patient no longer needs it and the hole closes off on its own after the tube is removed.

How long are patients on the ventilator after a tracheostomy is performed?

This depends on the patient's overall condition at the time the tracheostomy is performed. Two factors play a significant role in the patient's ventilator requirements: (1) whether the parts of the brain that control breathing are working and (2) the condition of the lungs. Portions of the brain stem and spinal cord help to control automatic breathing. Damage to these areas may result in the patient not being able to breathe without the use of the ventilator. This can be a permanent condition if these areas are irreversibly damaged, which can occur in severe neck injuries. More often the requirement for the ventilator stems from the patient's state of unconsciousness. Patients who are not awake enough may not breathe as much as is needed to get enough oxygen into the blood. Further, these patients often do not protect their airway in that oral secretions are allowed to enter the trachea (the airway leading to the lungs), which can lead to aspiration pneumonia.

Pneumonia and other types of damage to the lungs can make it difficult for the patient to get sufficient oxygen into the blood and to exhale enough carbon dioxide. If these conditions impair the normal function of the lungs, a ventilator may be necessary until the pneumonia can be treated with antibiotics or the damaged area recovers (the lung will typically recover from the pneumonia while areas of damaged brain often do not). Serial chest x-ray films and arterial blood gases are used to assess whether the lungs are recovering and doing an adequate job. Patients with pre-existing lung disease, such as emphysema or recurrent bronchitis, have a harder time than those without such problems. Older patients with head injury also have more difficulty overcoming the need for the ventilator because their breathing muscles are often not as strong as younger patients.

The placement of a tracheostomy facilitates the eventual removal of the ventilator. Similar to the endotracheal tube, it provides a pathway for the health care staff to suction out secretions and infectious material. It also acts to protect the airway in those patients who are unable to do so for themselves. The difficulty with endotracheal tubes is that if they are left in place for a prolonged period, they can cause tissue breakdown and swelling in the tissues around the airway. This can block the airway if the endotracheal tube is removed, resulting in the patient not being able to get air into the lungs. A tracheostomy solves this problem by bypassing the oral cavity (i.e., mouth). Also, patients can be given trial periods off the ventilator easily and safely with a tracheostomy in place. The ventilator tubing is simply removed and the patient breathes through the tracheostomy, which continues to protect the airway. If the patient still requires the ventilator, it can be reattached to the tracheostomy.

Patients on the ventilator without a tracheostomy in place must have the breathing tube removed to adequately assess whether the ventilator is necessary and whether the patient can protect the airway. Due to the swelling that may occur in the tissues around the endotracheal tube, this can be somewhat risky to the patient. Overall, a tracheostomy makes it easier and safer to wean patients off the ventilator. Depending on the condition of the lungs and the breathing centers within the brain, the period of time on the ventilator after the tracheostomy is placed can vary, but usually ranges from a few days to a week if all goes well.

Can the patient talk and eat with a tracheostomy in place?

Patients who no longer require the ventilator to breathe adequately and who recover some degree of consciousness may be able to eat. Such patients are often evaluated by a speech therapist, who makes sure that the patient is awake enough and physically able to both chew and swallow food properly. This is done to decrease the risk of aspiration. Because the swallowing tube, called the **esophagus,** is located behind the trachea, patients who have a tracheostomy in place can eat normally. However, those with an endotracheal tube in place cannot eat normally because this more bulky tube occupies a large portion of the mouth and throat, preventing the ability to adequately chew and swallow food.

Patients with tracheostomies can also talk. In order to talk normally, exhaled air from the lungs must be passed through the vocal cords. By manipulating the vocal cords, mouth, and tongue, sounds are made that we recognize as speech. The portions of the brain and brain stem that help control these areas must be intact for the speech produced to be comprehensible. If the speech centers in the brain are functioning normally, patients with a tracheostomy can produce speech by temporarily occluding the trach (covering the tracheostomy). This can easily be done with a fingertip. The air exhaled from the lungs is forced through the vocal cords instead of out the tracheostomy tube. The fingertip is then removed when it is time to take another breath, allowing the air to move through the tracheostomy tube into the lungs. With a little practice and speech therapy, patients with tracheostomies in place can often speak fairly well. There is also a device called the "talking trach" (pronounced trake [like bake]) that, in effect, does the same thing as temporarily occluding the trach at the time of exhalation. Patients with this device in place can breathe normally through the trach and talk when they want to without having to temporarily occlude the tracheostomy tube.

How do you close up a tracheostomy site? Will it leave a large scar?

As the patient improves and the tracheostomy is no longer necessary, it is removed in a step-by-step manner called "downsizing the trach." This process, in which the diameter of the tracheostomy tube is slowly reduced over time, allows the skin around the incision to gradually heal. Over time, the tracheostomy tubes are replaced with smaller and smaller tubes. As the diameter of the tracheostomy tube is decreased, the skin around the surgical hole begins to heal. As this occurs, the wound slowly begins to close. The hole remains open as long as a tracheostomy tube is in place but decreases in size as smaller tubes are used. Eventually, the tracheostomy can be completely removed. With time, the surgical hole left behind completely closes up; when this occurs, the patient breathes through the normal route. Most tracheostomies are placed just above the breast bone in the middle of the neck. The surgical incision made at the time of the surgery is approximately one inch long. While patients vary in terms of the amount of scar tissue that they develop at any wound site, the scar left behind from a tracheostomy is typically a small circle the size of a dime or quarter. In addition, due to the position of the incision, this area is usually not visible when the patient wears a shirt with a collar.

Why does the patient keep running a high temperature?

One of the jobs of the brain is to control all the automatic functions of the body. In fact, there is an entire part of the nervous system dedicated to taking care of these functions. These things include temperature regulation, breathing, digestion, heart function, and other functions that we never think about. We don't think about each breath we take, we just breathe because our body somehow knows to do it; this innate knowledge is a function of the **autonomic nervous system.** This system consists of specially designed nerves under the direct control of specific areas of the brain that take care of the day-to-day maintenance functions of the body. When the brain is injured, its ability to take care of these normal functions may be impaired. Temperature regulation is one aspect of this system that is commonly affected. The brain loses its ability to work as the body's thermostat and allows the temperature to go out of control. Temperatures as high as 40° C or 105° F are not uncommon. Unfortunately, high temperatures may also be a sign of infection. Any patient with persistently high temperatures must have frequent urine, sputum and blood tests to make sure an infectious source for the fever is not being overlooked.

Why does the patient need arm and leg splints?

Patients with head injury often have problems with increased tone in their muscles. The nerves and muscles in the body are directly related to one another. When a nerve is injured, the muscle that it supplies undergoes specific changes. Every muscle in the body is under the direct control of a nerve and every nerve in the body is intimately linked to the brain. Patients with injured brains often develop changes in their arms and legs. These changes result from involuntary muscle contractions caused by changes in the nervous **innervation** to the muscles. Basically, the brain injury adversely affects the signals traveling from the brain through the nerves into the muscles. Without the proper signals, the muscles will not act properly. They begin to slowly contract and this can lead to permanent deformities if not treated. By applying leg, wrist, and hand splints, the muscles are held in their proper alignment. The splints act to replace the normal, proper nerve impulses that are not being sent to the muscles because of the injury. As the brain heals, it is possible to regain near-normal signals to the muscles and the need for the splints no longer remains.

What are the pneumatic stockings for?

Pneumatic air stockings are placed on the legs of almost every patient who will be bedridden for an extended period of time. These patients are at high risk for developing blood clots in their legs. Blood clots, also known as DVTs, can be a serious threat to the patient's health. The clots may come loose and travel through the bloodstream, getting lodged in the heart or lungs. This often causes serious problems with respiration and may even be fatal.

These blood clots or DVTs can form when the blood flow through the legs is slower than normal. When a patient is bedridden, the leg muscles do not go through a normal daily exercise cycle. In healthy people, the pumping of blood through the leg veins is done by the continuous contraction of the leg muscles. Just walking around produces enough pumping action to prevent blood clots from forming. Patients who are bedridden do not move their legs enough to create adequate pumping. Thus the blood pools in their legs and, as the blood collects, it begins to clot. These clots can produce leg swelling and pain, but the real danger is when a piece of the clot breaks off and travels through the veins to the lungs. Here it can become trapped and block blood flow into the lungs. Without blood flow, the lungs cannot function and, when the lungs fail to work, the heart stops and the patient can die. Even placement on a ventilator may not save the patient because the lungs must have constant blood flow to perform gas exchange. The ventilator can send fresh oxygenated air into the lungs but, without blood flowing through to take the oxygen to the rest of the body, the patient will die.

This blockage of the lung's blood supply is known as a **pulmonary embolism.** In this situation, the patient must be placed immediately on powerful blood thinners or taken for emergency surgery. In the time it takes to bring the patient to the operating room and prepare them for surgery, it is often too late. The use of blood thinners is effective if the pulmonary embolism is relatively small and if they are started right away. One problem with head injury patients is that thinning their blood is often dangerous because of the brain injury. Thinning the blood can cause bleeding in the brain so it is not always an option in treating DVTs in serious head injury cases.

The best option for treating DVTs and pulmonary embolism is prevention. This is done with pneumatic air stockings and small doses of heparin (a blood-thinning drug) injected under the skin. The use of heparin lowers the risk of DVTs but does not increase the risk of intracranial hemorrhages. The pneumatic stockings are essentially balloons that are wrapped around the patient's legs; these are then hooked up to a machine that sequentially inflates and then deflates them. This creates the pumping action on the muscles in the legs that is necessary to propel the blood through the veins. Pneumatic stockings and heparin dramatically lower the incidence of blood clot formation.

CHAPTER

9

❧·❧

Prognosis and Outcomes: What the Future Holds

The most fundamental question is what type of recovery and function can be expected from a patient with head injury. Unfortunately, there is no simple equation to apply or test that can be performed to accurately predict the actual outcome. No two patients are the same, and while one can do extremely well, another, with the same amount of injury, may do very poorly. Patients who might be expected to do poorly can surprise doctors and do well; conversely, those who are expected to do well may do poorly. There is without question a certain element of the unknown, as there is in many aspects of medicine. In general, a combination of factors determine the likely outcome for a particular patient. These include the location and severity of the initial injury, the presence of any other associated injuries, the clinical course after the accident, and the patient's state of health prior to the accident. Obviously, the more the patient must overcome, in terms of the injury's severity and complications related to that injury, the less favorable the outcome.

Donna: *We were always asking, "Do you think Sharon knows we're here at least?" and "Do you think she's ever going to come out* *of this?" Some doctors and nurses said, "You know, you've got a long road ahead of you." I wanted to know if she was going to die. And, at the beginning, of course, they couldn't answer that, but after a few days in the ICU, they said they didn't think she would die, but that it was just a matter of waiting and seeing what happened.*

Having discussed the element of uncertainty surrounding actual outcomes from head injury, there are some fundamental concepts, based on extensive research, that are generally thought to be true. Little can be done for the brain injury that occurs at the time of impact in an accident. Contrary to prior beliefs, however, the patient's fate is not sealed at the time of the accident. While the injury occurring at the time of the accident may be permanent, the injury process continues for days after the accident. It is the disruption of this injury process that is the focus of all treatments for head injury. The idea is to prevent further injury by keeping the injury process to a minimum and to begin healing the injury that has already occurred. Sometimes this results in a successful outcome. Other times the initial injury is so severe that little can be done to help the patient. Those with very severe head injury often die before they reach the hospital.

It seems that the type of recovery and the function that the patient will attain are largely dependent on the severity of the initial injury. Those patients with more severe initial injuries tend to do worse than those with less severe injury. Other factors that play a role in the likely outcome are the patient's age, the type of injury incurred, and the location of the injury. On average, patients older than 40 years of age do worse than those who are younger. Patients younger than 20 years of age appear to do the best, all other aspects being equal.

Ellen: *I expected Steve not to live, I really did. After losing his father to the same type of accident, it just seemed inevitable. I guess I was trying to prepare myself for the worst. At that point, I didn't even care if there was brain damage, if he was going to be different. I just* *wanted him to survive. But my son made a remarkable recovery. He literally walked out of the ICU, which the staff couldn't believe. They said nobody does that. He walked out the door. Well, of course, they had to put him in a wheelchair, but he did incredibly well. They think it was because he was young and healthy with a strong will to live and a lot to live for. Steve doesn't remember anything about that day, which has been hard for him. He has questions that may never be answered.*

The only real physical difference now is that one eye is slightly lower than the other. I see it because I'm his mother, but no one else would notice. Before the accident, he spent hours in front of the mirror styling his hair. In the hospital they shaved his head and his hair grew back really strange, but he thinks it's great. He gets in the shower, washes it, and shakes it a bit! He has a whole different attitude, real easy come, easy go. The accident taught him something about the value of life—something many never learn.

He starts junior college in January, just 6 months behind schedule. They said we could expect some problems when he starts school. His concentration might be off and he might get frustrated. We don't know because we haven't been on that course yet. He has a job, though, and he's doing great. Everything seems fine.

A large-group study,[1] conducted at a number of hospitals, has been performed that looked at the outcomes of 746 patients with head injury, with severe head injury defined as a **Glasgow Coma Score** or **GCS** of 3 to 8. In terms of outcome, patients can be roughly divided into two main groups: those with favorable outcomes and those with unfavorable outcomes. Patients with a favorable outcome are generally considered to be those who can return to normal daily activities with little or no assistance; patients with unfavorable outcomes are those who die, remain in a permanent coma, called a **persistent vegetative state,** or those with severe disabilities requiring continual care, typically in some sort of institution. Of the 746 patients in the study, just less than half (42%) had a favorable outcome. Patients with a GCS of 9 or more did better, with 61% having a favorable outcome.

Donna: *Sharon was in rehabilitation from October until the end of February. She woke up in November. It was weird when she woke up. You don't really know what to expect until you experience something like this. It wasn't just like, "Oh, I'm awake now." It began with little signs. She started nodding first and then blowing kisses! The nurse blew her a kiss and she blew a kiss back. And so for a while, we played games blowing kisses and stuff. Then she started moving her arms and legs up and down, not really trying to do anything, just moving like she was nervous or restless. What made us realize that she was really out of the coma was when she started talking. She was still in a level of a coma, probably still a 2 or a 3. She didn't know for sure who I was, she called me Katy (her daughter) sometimes. But I didn't care. I was so happy to hear her speak and I felt like she was really making good progress.*

She's home now. We are all so proud of her. She can walk with a cane. If she ran into an acquaintance she hadn't seen in a year or so, and who didn't know all she had been through, they might be taken aback because she's different, she's not like she was. Sometimes, though, she does or says something that makes me think, "Yeah, that's my Sharon." Little phrases or just looks or gestures that I recognize as her . . .

The anniversary of the accident was a difficult day, but when I think about it, I think, "Boy, just a year ago, this is what she was, and look at her now. She's doing things, she's reading, she can walk, she's alive."

We've been told that, within the first 6 months to a year, patients make a lot of progress and then it slows down. That has been our experience. But she's still making progress. My other sister, who visits every 3 or 4 weeks, sees improvements in Sharon that those of us who see her everyday miss altogether.

Her husband asks me if I think she's getting better, or if I've noticed that she's really trying to get into conversations. For awhile, she just kind of sat in a daze most of the time and really didn't join in conversations. I had a graduation party for her son and she was really glad that everybody was there, even people from out of town, but she wasn't participating much. I hated to see that but I was just thankful that she was here at all. She still doesn't talk as much as she used to, but she does tell me things, and it's almost like having my sister back.

The study also reviewed the incidence of surgery and the outcomes related to these operations. Approximately one third of the patients required surgery (37% of the total 746 patients). The most common reason for surgery in these patients was for a **subdural hematoma** (58% of the patients who required surgery), followed by contusions (26%) and **epidural hematomas** (16%). Among these three groups, patients with epidural hematomas had the highest percentage of favorable outcomes (47% of these patients who underwent surgery). Patients who required surgery for a subdural hematoma had the highest number of deaths and the least percentage of favorable recoveries (50% of these patients died and only 14% had a favorable outcome). Age also appeared to play a factor in the outcomes. In the group of patients requiring surgery, 64% of the patients older than 40 years of age died, while less than one third (28%) of the patients under 40 years of age died.[1] While this is just one study, it examined a large number of patients treated at different medical centers. Therefore, while there are unique circumstances with every patient, these results are likely close to being representative of what to expect in severe head injury patients.

Sarah: *Eight days after the operation Jim was off the respirator. The breathing tube was removed 12 days later. He moved to rehabilitation on day 16 and still didn't know where he was. He could move his arms but he didn't have balance yet, so he was in a wheelchair . . .*

Following a head injury they told me it would be up to 2 years to recover. I thought, "Gosh, that's a long time," when I thought of someone sitting in a hospital and their whole life stopping. Two years was just unacceptable. In my mind I only thought, "He'll be better in six months." I was always optimistic.

The accident was a year and a half ago. Jim's still not perfect, but he's wonderful. He's home now. We have a farm and his dad has a farm, so he's been busy. . . . He's up and around and, to look at him, you think he is fine, you never suspect that he had had such a traumatic experience.

The only residual thing is that his personality is not as relaxed, and I don't know if that will change. Hopefully, once he gets back to working and feels more comfortable with himself. Early on, his moods were awful and we were told that was typical with people who have had head injuries. They can be really aggressive or upset. It was especially hard for the kids to understand. Even now, Joshua occasionally says he's just not the same.

It could have been a lot worse. Anybody can always think that. It could always be worse. The main thing that helped Jim and I keep things in perspective was when we went back to the hospital for follow-up visits and saw all the people in the waiting room. We thought, "Oh, we're doing real good." We realized we were among the lucky ones.

He's back to doing physical things now. Last harvest he drove a tandem truck and did all kinds of farm work. I'm confident that he could also do his regular job but his employer won't allow him to return to work while he is taking antiseizure medication.

❧ COMMONLY ASKED QUESTIONS ❧

Is the patient going to die?

It is very difficult to predict a patient's individual outcome, particularly in dealing with the residual function that will be present after recovery from the injury. Those patients with more severe head injuries and those who are older are more likely to die than younger, less severely injured patients. Additional injuries to other parts of the body, particularly the heart and lungs, increase the likelihood of death, as do other medical problems that may have been present before the injury or as a result of being in the **intensive care unit** or **ICU** for a prolonged period of time. These include severe pneumonia, blood clots that travel to the lungs **(pulmonary embolism),** serious infection (particularly in the brain), and heart, lung, and kidney disease. The patients who typically do *not* survive the injury are those who have very severe head injury with extremely elevated **intracranial pressures** or **ICPs,** difficulty in getting enough oxygen into the blood (usually from lung damage or extensive infection), and those with multiple injuries to other organs, such as the heart, lung, liver and spleen.

How long will the patient remain in a coma?

Unfortunately, there is no test or examination that can determine how long someone will be unconscious. Patients with severe head injuries tend to remain unconscious for longer periods of time than those with less severe injuries. Further, as the patient's brain recovers, the "wake up process" is usually gradual, not sudden as if awakening from sleep. This period of "awakening" after head injury can vary from just a few days or up to several months. Again, the more severe the injury, the longer it takes to recover. Depending on the circumstances of the injury and the response that the patient makes to the various treatments, it is possible that the patient may never regain consciousness and may remain in a **persistent vegetative state.** Physicians rely on studies and trends to make general assessments on the likelihood of recovery. If the patient shows signs of improvement, and the improvement appears to continue while in the hospital, it is more likely that the patient will continue that trend even after being discharged, as opposed to a patient who shows no signs of recovery over a prolonged period of time (i.e., weeks or months). As always, there are exceptions to the rule. Patients who show no signs of recovery or have been completely unconscious for months can improve, but this is definitely not the norm.

Will the patient wake up?

There is no way to predict whether a patient will eventually wake up. Even more important, if the patient does wake up, the type of function and abilities that will be present is somewhat in doubt. Patients who show signs of waking up while in the hospital within the first week or two tend to have an increased chance of waking up completely compared to those who do not. This wake-up process can take weeks or months and, despite a seemingly rapid initial improvement, it may plateau and then begin to improve again. Family members dealing with head injury should keep in mind that this recovery process, whether it be waking up or recovering function (such as moving, talking, and thinking), typically can take from months to years.

Can you compare other patients with the same head injury and tell me how well you can expect a patient to do?

This is difficult because the outcome from a head injury is dependent on many different variables. While two patients may have roughly the same type and location of injury, one may do very well while the other patient does poorly. These differences may be for many reasons, including the age of the patient, any other complications that may present, and the overall health of the patient before the accident. Patients with less severe injuries tend to do better than those who have more involved injuries. Complications, such as uncontrollable elevated ICPs, infection, bleeding problems leading to larger bruises within the brain, periods in which there isn't enough oxygen in the blood **(hypoxia),** or the combination of a serious spinal cord injury, decrease the chances for a good recovery. More complications can lead to more damage within the brain. Although two patients may start out with the similar injuries, one may end up with considerably more damage than the other because of these complications. Unfortunately, there is no accurate way to predict which, if any, of these complications will occur in any given patient.

In general, patients who are talking (even though not necessarily making sense), moving around purposefully (such that the movements are directed toward achieving a goal), and have either close to normal or controllable ICPs do better than those patients who do not have these characteristics. The trend that the patient displays is also an important indicator of the expected outcome. Patients who begin to show signs of improvement early on, such as beginning to move more purposefully, or those in whom the ICPs

208 • I The Acute Phase

are beginning to drop, tend to do better than those who continue to exhibit more **posturing** types of movement (automatic movements in response to a stimuli) or have increasing ICPs.

What is a vegetative state? Will the patient remain in a vegetative state? How can you tell?

A vegetative state is a situation in which the patient displays absolutely no higher cortical functions (i.e., brain functions, such as communication, purposeful movements, or evidence of thought) but the brain stem continues to function. The patient breathes, has normal pupillary activity, and may chew and even swallow. None of these actions is under the patient's conscious control because the patient is not awake; although the eyes may be open, the brain itself is not functioning. The higher cortical centers that enable us to think, feel, and have emotions are no longer working.

Long-term survival in a vegetative state is uncommon, only about 1% to 2% of patients survive for any significant period of time. It is difficult to give a realistic prognosis after the first 24 hours of vegetative symptoms. Some patients may be in a vegetative state but improve rapidly. Signs of steady improvement may reflect recovery from the injury, but these improvements, if they are going to occur, usually manifest relatively early after the initial brain insult. Many studies have been done to predict prognosis for patients in a vegetative state. All of them show that prognosis for patients who remain in a vegetative state for more than 2 weeks is extremely poor. None of the patients studied was ever able to resume meaningful activity or even take part in any form of basic human interaction.

1. Marshall LF, Gautille T, Klauber MR, et al. The outcome of severe closed head injury. J Neurosurg 75:S28-S36, 1991.

CHAPTER
10

Emotional Reactions and
Coping Strategies

Elisabeth Price, Ph.D., M.A.
Sr. Ann Johnston, O.P.
Rev. Gregory Kirsch, M.Div., M.A.

The family arrives at the hospital and waits ... After waiting hours for news about her injured child, a mother in the emergency department says, "This day has changed our lives forever. Can anything good come of this terrible event?" The answer is that although the disaster cannot be undone, many good things can and will happen in the future. Meanwhile, the entire family has to go through the initial shock and grief caused by the head injury. How they do this can affect the well-being of the family and the future of the patient. The initial period of waiting is characterized by fear, anguish, uncertainty, and suspense. Everyone needs to make use of any and all help that is available. At this time, emotional, physical, and spiritual needs often merge and can be alleviated by the caring presence of others and their offers of support and help.

Donna: Sharon's daughter was actually the first one to get to the hospital because she worked at a hotel close by. When she heard her mother was there, she became hysterical just like me. We were all just totally out of it. But the scariest part was when we got to the hospital, they took us to what they called the "quiet room" for families who have a major injury, and a chaplain or some other counselor is present.

We just wanted to know if Sharon would be okay, but, of course, no one knew. . . . It was so chaotic . . . so we all went to the quiet room and waited and cried.

THE COMPLEX EMOTIONS AND NEEDS OF THE FAMILY

When people first hear about traumatic brain injury in someone they love, guilt, denial, anger, fear, and shock are normal, even predictable reactions. It is important to acknowledge that almost any reaction is acceptable as long as it does no harm to the self or others. People may need some assistance in containing their emotions. Privacy and the support of others may help.

Everyone affected must be allowed to feel their emotions and to express them in a healthy way. The first instinct may be to disbelieve that the injury is really serious. "He's going to be okay, isn't he?" When they realize it is serious, many people need to cry, wail, or even scream. It is important to let this happen so that emotions are released. However, people should avoid working themselves into a frenzy, as this will only add to their distress. They may be able to calm down with a touch on the shoulder or a hug (if appropriate) and supportive phrases such as, "Calm down, we will help you through this" or "Take it easy, we are here with you." The first response to this is sometimes, "Leave me alone." or "Get away from me," and some people may need time to collect themselves before being able to accept the support of others. It is important not to offer any false reassurance, such as saying, "Everything's going to be fine," when this is not the case. Nor is it helpful to tell people to "Be strong!" at the moment they feel that their life has fallen apart. It is appropriate to reassure adults that their strength and maturity are still intact, that they will eventually find ways to deal with the situation, and that others are ready and able to help.

Donna: *I needed some escape from the stress. I worked out just about everyday. As many days as I could, I did at least a half-hour of exercise, go for a walk or something. I could never go back to the exercise class I used to attend at the YMCA. Sharon and I always went there together and we really had a good time. Sometimes, if I didn't feel like going, Sharon went anyway. She was kind of a motivator for me. "C'mon, let's go, you'll feel better!" she'd say. I miss that.*

The first couple of weeks or so I still had a hard time accepting what had happened. I thought, "Oh, I'm going to wake up," and "This is just a bad dream." Then I realized life has to go on. I went and did something with the kids for the day, take them somewhere, or do something with my husband. But I never really stopped thinking about it.

I appreciate every little thing that Sharon can do now. I realize how much we all take for granted.

The Stress of Uncertainty

During the acute phase of severe head injury the patient is usually unconscious. Family members, friends, and bystanders anxiously await the signs of any awakening, awareness of self and others, and then orientation to place and time. The injured person's spiritual needs as consciousness returns are for reassurance of safety and security, the caring presence of loved ones, and hope that the situation will improve. Family members and friends often instinctively respond to those needs with their own desires to communicate and express love and hope. Some may need to be reminded, in their own great distress, that the injured person is not able at this time to meet their emotional needs, and that they must turn to others for emotional support. It is especially difficult to see the many symptoms of head injury in someone who is very close or has been a source of strength in the past.

Donna: *In order for me to cope with the emotions, I think just going there and being with her were the most important things. I read to her a lot. I remember bringing the newspaper one day and when I began* *reading it aloud the nurse, Flo, said, "There probably isn't anything good in there! Maybe you could find something more up-beat!" So most of the time I read cards and a book of poems my boss had given me. I also read the Bible to her. Reading aloud made me feel like I was doing something for Sharon. I think we both benefited from it.*

We also prayed a lot. Actually, sometimes I felt like I was praying too much because every chance I had, I prayed, "Just let her be okay."

A head injury of someone close is one of the greatest stressors individuals and family members can experience. The staff caring for the injured person, witnesses to the event, and even others, such as distant acquaintances or people sharing the space in the waiting room, are also affected by this stress. A loss has occurred, the extent of which may not be fully known for some time. There is often a feeling that if it could happen to the person concerned, it could happen to anyone, and feelings of insecurity are aroused in everyone who hears about it. How and why the loss happened in a particular case may not be clear and may, in some cases, never be known. Dealing with uncertainty is one of the most difficult spiritual tasks posed by head injury. For others, knowing what happened, or who is to blame, if there is such a person, may not provide any resolution of tension. It may rouse more anger or present additional issues that are difficult to deal with. Seeking out the support of others is very important for family members and friends.

Sarah: I have lots of sisters and Jim has a big family, so we had plenty of help. I really had to rely on my family and friends. . . . My advice is to willingly accept whatever friends, family, and community offer, whether it be fast-food, childcare, or gas. We had an outpouring of generosity from our neighbors and the businesses in our small town.

It can be difficult to admit to any kind of hardship and accept help . . . It is important to overcome your pride and take whatever they are offering because it can only make you feel better. I was overwhelmed by everyone's generosity, it just made me feel that everyone cares and I was loved.

Fear

The basic emotional response in those experiencing a loved one's head injury is fear, not only for the life of the injured person, but also about changes in personality and identity that have been the basis of the relationships of that person with others. Fear of loss of love and pleasure join the immediate fear of death. Resentment and irritation at loss of peace of mind and disturbance of normal routine may accompany the fear and even be used as an emotional barrier against feeling the full brunt of the fear. Depending on the cause of the injury, other very strong feelings may arise, such as anger, guilt, blame, desire for retaliation, or desire to punish oneself.

> **Ellen:** *The chaplain came and sat with us and that helped us focus on priorities. I don't know what we would have done if Steve had died. I think I would have gone completely out of my mind. I really do. But I have the other kids to think about, too. My mom and dad kept saying, "You're gonna pull through this, you're gonna." "Not if something happens, Mom, not this time, I've already lost a husband this way. I can't lose a son, too. I'm not gonna take it this time." I went through the whole, "I'll never go to church again," thing . . . but that's normal I think. It was unbelievably bizarre. That's the best way to describe it. I'll never forget that part of my life for as long as I live. You would think it would be a blur but . . . my emotions were nuts. I was in there with all my friends, I was laughing, and all of a sudden I found myself crying. My emotions were completely out of whack, mainly because I was exhausted.*

Anger

Many people express their strong feelings by asking why the injury happened. The question may take many forms, depending on the identity of the injured person and the circumstances of the injury, ranging from, "Why did this happen to someone so young and innocent?" to "Why could the recklessness or evil that caused this not be stopped?" The event may seem unjust. If a cause is evident, such as risky or aggressive behavior, whether by the person injured or someone else, the outcome still may not seem reasonable. If a criminal act or gross irresponsibility is involved, feelings of outrage may be even stronger.

Feelings of helplessness may also trigger depression or anger. Once the injured person has been brought to the hospital, there is little or nothing family members and friends can do to contribute to the actual medical treatment in the acute phase. The initial rescue of the injured person may have taken place out of sight and without the knowledge of the family members. Having little or no control over the trauma happening to a loved one can cause people to feel powerless and frustrated.

There may be other reasons to feel angry and/or depressed, such as if others have been injured in the same incident, if there is extensive property damage, and if criminal charges are being pressed. Every head injury has its own complex scenario. In addition, there may have been difficulties in the patient's life before the injury. Relationships with family members and friends may not always have been smooth and this increases the complexity of emotions felt in relation to the injury.

Ellen: I stayed overnight at the hospital. Fortunately, I had a lot of support. My mother and father live nearby and they and my brothers, sisters, and neighbors were just unbelievable. I never had to worry about the other children and the day-to-day concerns.

It was the hardest, I think, for my younger son. He and Steve were inseparable. They were 17 and 18 years old at the time. He was a mess. He couldn't stand to go home without Steve there. It was also very difficult for my husband because he was like their dad and he was so shook up about this. The younger kids kind of went on with their lives. They went to school and their normal activities . . . but it was so hard on everybody in the family.

Supporting Children and Teens

In the case of children, it is important to express loving concern and the assurance of continuing adult support. Young children need simple concrete facts to help them understand, such as, "Daddy is badly hurt. The doctors are trying to get him well." Unfortunately, the answer to most questions, such as, "Is he going to get well? When is he going to get well?" is "We don't know yet." An attempt to deny the uncertainties and fears of the adults around them will confuse children, because they will sense they are being deceived. Children should be supported by the assurance that the adults in their lives love them, will stay with them, and will help them, no matter what happens. For young children no long explanations are necessary; usually they ask for the information when they are ready to hear it. Sometimes they overhear remarks made by adults that may need interpretation or correction, for example, forecasts of the future that may or may not come about, or assigning blame that may or may not be appropriate. A child can usually face uncertainty about what is going to happen, provided that plenty of love and assurance is available in the here and now.

> **Ellen:** *I regret my initial reaction when I heard about the accident. I lost it. I've never reacted that way in a situation, but I just . . . and it really scared the younger boys. David, my 13-year-old son, kept saying, "Is he going to be all right?" and I kept screaming, "No, he's not, no, he's not." I just assumed he wouldn't. I look back at that and I think, "Why did I lose control like that?" Those poor little kids.*
>
> *As I said, Tony and Steve were as close as two brothers could be. They were inseparable. And Tony is a very quiet young man; he keeps everything inside. We were worried about him and how he was handling the situation.*
>
> *He was literally sick. He wasn't eating, didn't want to go to school. He's a straight A student, but he just couldn't cope with the idea. I made him go back to school because he had exams.*

That was the hardest. Oh, that poor kid. I really worried just as much about the other kids as I did about my son in the hospital. You don't know which one . . .

Older children and teenagers may ask many questions. It is important to acknowledge their need for information and to provide it if possible. They need many of the same types of support that can help adults. If possible, they also need to process their feelings with their peer group, often in the context of activities that have nothing to do with what is going on in their own family at the moment.

Sarah: *There was a lot of scheduling and coordinating in terms of taking care of the kids and keeping things going on the farm. I have three children, the youngest was only a year old at the time. It was hard, they just wanted me home. . . . It's important to keep the family going, the kids won't let everything stop. The soccer games, parties, everything needs to go on as near to normal as possible.*

COPING METHODS
During the Shock Stage of Grief

People of all ages respond in widely different ways. Some people are stunned into silence when receiving the news. They need to be given time to take in the situation quietly in their own way. Some people may repeat the same sentence over and over again, expressing a first reaction such as, "I told her not to do that!" "Why? Why? Why?" or "Mother will never forgive me!" Some may need to walk around, pace the floor, or go outside. All need the space and privacy to have these reactions. Someone may need to look out for their safety until they have regained their self-possession. If the hospital has not already provided this, ask if there is a more private space where people will not be exposed to the further stress of strangers' observing their grief. If no separate space is available, it may be possible to create a circle of privacy by rearranging chairs or otherwise grouping together. If the first person arrives at the hospital alone, the hospital staff should arrange for someone to provide that person with emotional support. That someone may well be the hospital chaplain, who will assist in calling other family members and friends and notifying clergy or church members who could be of help at this time.

Role of the Hospital Chaplain

When people find the hospital chaplain present, they are sometimes afraid that the patient is dead or is going to die. While chaplains do provide support in the case of death, they are also called for assistance in many other situations. Some people find it helpful simply to tell the chaplain the story of the event leading to the brain injury and to talk about the injured person. People may find relief in explaining what this injury may mean to them and to their families. It is always appropriate to ask the chaplain to pray, to read from the Bible, or to bless the injured person and the family members. The chaplain can help with sacramental needs, such as the Anointing of the Sick for Roman Catholics, Episcopalians, and others for whom this practice is significant. If the family is not comfortable with formal religious practices or prayers said out loud, it is entirely appropriate to make use of the chaplain's assistance with emotional and spiritual needs that are not seen as specifically religious. Professional hospital chaplains are trained to assist people with any religious affiliation or none. They accept and respect the spirituality and personal beliefs of everyone and help people use their own faith or system of beliefs to further their health and well-being.

The hospital chaplain can also assist with facilitating communication between hospital staff and family and friends who, for practical reasons, cannot always have access to the treatment area while the patient is in unstable or critical condition. Health care staff are trained to provide for the emotional needs of families, but their first concern must always be for the patient's treatment. In a situation of great uncertainty, the people waiting feel a desperate need for information. The chaplain will try to obtain and provide as much information as possible. In the absence of a hospital chaplain, someone else on the medical team should take the responsibility of keeping family members and friends informed. If a larger group gathers, it is helpful if one person acts as the spokesperson for everyone. This is frequently the next-of-kin, but if that person is in too great distress, someone else can help by taking on that role at least temporarily.

The Waiting Room Scenario: Filling the Void

Once initial emotional reactions have been accepted, it is possible to take practical steps to meet some of the needs that might arise while waiting in the hospital. Family members may wish to keep a journal or diary to record thoughts, feelings, and experiences, the visitors who come, the telephone calls received, and the flowers, gifts, and cards that arrive. This information not only helps process the history of this time, but may be greatly valued later by a patient who has lost all sense of the time spent in the hospital.

> **Ellen:** *I kept two journals, one that I wrote in everyday with the medical progress and so on, and another journal for people who came to visit. It was really neat for Steve to read later, because all of his friends and everybody wrote such nice things.*
>
> *I definitely recommend keeping a journal, both for yourself and to share with the patient later. I think it probably helped me more than the patient. It was very important for my 17-year-old son. He wrote in it every single day.*
>
> *It was really difficult to keep my act together for my kids, but I had to try because they were falling apart too. My poor little guys were worried. They didn't know what was going to happen. The journal was an outlet for our feelings.*

To help you deal with your situation, make a list of all your worries. You can sort these concerns into things you cannot change, things you can do something about, and information you need to obtain. Make a list of questions you need answered by doctors, nurses, and the social worker, and then ask each person whose help you need to set aside time for you to answer your questions as fully as possible. Each should tell you when your questions go beyond his or her expertise and refer you to someone who can help.

> **Sarah:** *Everyone is worried and emotional. Other family members may say something without realizing how it sounds. They don't mean to be insensitive, it's just that they're frightened. Right after the accident, someone made a comment, "I hope he's not retarded when he wakes up." I couldn't believe what I was hearing. And when a nurse mentioned a chaplain, another family member said, "Oh, we want to wait for a Catholic." I nearly lost it, in front of the whole family! Now we can look back and laugh, but at the time it just wasn't funny.*
>
> *When dealing with somebody who is stressed out, watch out! Think about what you're saying. And try not to be hurt or offended by what others say to you.*

You can also make a list of practical help you may need, such as driving, baby-sitting, shopping, laundry, and other errands, and ask those friends and relatives who have offered to help to do something specific for you. This exercise serves two purposes. First, you will have peace of mind that things are not falling through the cracks. Second, being able to help may also provide a positive outlet for friends' feelings. Some people would like to help right away while you are in the waiting room. They can be asked to pray, but they can also do little practical things like bringing in some hard candy, a box of Saltine crackers, or rolls of coins for the pay phone.

If you feel too tired to get organized, ask someone else who has more energy to help you start on these plans. If no family or friends are available or able to do this, it is appropriate to ask the hospital chaplain for help. Chaplains and other hospital staff have seen many people go through times like this and can offer helpful suggestions and ideas. Chaplains can be asked for assistance in the hospital with obtaining blankets, pillows, food and drink, a place to stay, and other practical matters.

Some people feel that their presence in the hospital is needed around the clock to ensure that everything goes well. This is not realistic because everyone else in the family has important needs, and the medical staff will watch over the patient when family members are needed elsewhere.

> **Ellen:** I didn't go home until I was pushed out by the nurse and then by the other family members. I just told them, "As soon as he opens his eyes and he knows that I'm here, then I can leave. I think it was about the ninth day that I said, "Okay, I can go home now and come back later."

It is extremely hard work to take on the task of organizing the family members in the midst of disaster, and it is very tiring to experience the stress and emotions involved in trauma. Everyone needs to get plenty of rest, eat regular meals with healthy foods, and get some exercise. Family life must be continued as normally as possible because those not injured still need support and even extra attention to calm their fears. If at all possible, people need to sleep at night in their own beds. Ask others to help organize shifts of people staying at the hospital and people responsible for keeping the household going. People are usually glad to help as long as they know exactly what is needed. Often, more resources for help are available than those that immediately come to mind. Besides your family, neighbors, church and other organization members, coworkers, and parents of children's friends may be glad to offer support. They realize that the situation is unusual and calls for extra help. Many families find that they can support and be supported by others in the waiting room at the hospital who are experiencing similar problems.

Ellen: My heart goes out to other families suffering through this experience. I remember coming in one time and there was a whole bunch of people in the waiting room. My heart just broke. I was ecstatic that day because they were moving Steve out of the ICU and we had a camera and were taking pictures of each other. All of a sudden I thought, "Oh, my God, we're being so insensitive to these other people. We shouldn't be doing this." But nobody reacted like that, nobody; they were happy for us. Families become close to other families.

Connecting With the Injured Person

The injured person is everyone's main concern. It is possible to give love by being present at the bedside for short visits. The health care staff will tell you when it is appropriate to stimulate the patient and when it is not. Injury of the nervous system can lead to oversensitivity to stimulus and then visits have to be made very quietly and quickly. When the patient can tolerate contact with family and friends, there are many creative ways to keep in touch. Check with the nurse concerning what you may bring into the intensive care unit or ICU. Flowers are not usually allowed, but often balloons are permitted, and cards, drawings, pictures, and messages can be taped to the wall or to a mirror. Tapes of favorite music can be played. In the case of young patients, friends who cannot visit may be able to tape a message. The sounds of home, such as a beloved dog barking, a baby crying, children playing, or someone practicing a musical instrument, can also be taped. Whether the patient is responsive or not, all the news from home and about family and friends can be told. Both the patient and family members need to know that life outside the hospital is still going on. Each family finds its unique ways of trying to communicate with the patient. Teenage friends or siblings may want to keep a journal of their own to share with each other and the injured person later. This can pass the time in the waiting room or during periods of loneliness.

Finding Psychological and Spiritual Support in the Hospital

There are more ways to help those in the waiting room spend time positively. Often hospitals offer support groups for family members of critically ill patients. It can be worthwhile to make the effort to attend. Under stress, it can be hard to concentrate and many people say that they cannot meditate or pray, although they want to. Remember that short prayers are just as valid as long ones. If you cannot summon the energy to pray, let others do it for you. Help with prayer is readily available from the hospital chaplain, your own clergy, friends from your church, and sometimes from other unexpected sources, such as hospital staff, volunteers, and others in the waiting room. Prayer does not have to be formulated in traditional words (although Bibles should be available throughout the hospital and certainly from the chaplains' office). Try a simple slow, deep breathing technique where you imagine yourself breathing in love, or courage, or peace, and breathing out fear, or resentment, or despair. This will help you relax. Visualization techniques can be helpful. See yourself creating a ball of energy from the sun, the moon, and the earth and then send it to the one you love inside the ICU. Or, if you are concerned about others in your family traveling a long distance to visit the hospital, create a ball of energy to send to them. Visit the hospital chapel for a change of scene. Feel all the heartfelt prayers that have been made there in the past and let your own hopes and fears join those of countless others in the human family. Record your spiritual journey in a journal. Sometimes, it helps not only to write feelings down, but to read and reread them.

> *Ellen: We did a lot of praying. It really helped. More than anything it was the love and support of family members and friends and prayers that got me through this experience. But, it wasn't all sitting around and praying. Some people probably thought we were crazy, but occasionally we laughed and told jokes. We had to. It helps release tension and life has to go on.*

Friends and family members were really there for me. I came home, the place was spotless, and there was a meal on the table. It was friends and family who pulled me through. I would have gone nuts especially that month of June. It was hell.

Every now and then I think about the accident. It pops into my mind when I least expect it. My eyes just well up with tears and I start to cry and think, "Oh, my God, how did I get through that?" I didn't realize how strong I could be.

But don't be strong by yourself. Let people help you. You can't do it by yourself. You may want to, but you can't. I was fine, but I was pretty obstinate with some of the nurses who were trying to be helpful and send me home to sleep. When I kept refusing, one nurse said, "You're gonna be right there in that bed next to him if you don't get your act together." I said, "Fine." Later I apologized for being so mean." She was a neat lady and said she understood.

Taking Care of Your Own Health

Some hospital waiting rooms have no windows. Make sure you see daylight from time to time. Take walks outside, if possible, or inside the hospital if you cannot go out. If you can, leave the hospital for meals. If eating is difficult, try foods that are easy to swallow and not too rich or spicy. If a need for energy makes you overeat, try walking or jogging to stimulate your circulation instead. Rather than using harmful stimulants, such as caffeine and alcohol, find someone to talk to, or ask someone to rub your back. If nausea, diarrhea, sleeplessness, trembling and other physical symptoms persist over several days, ask your own doctor for help in controlling these.

Sarah: I had to keep going to work, and it was actually good for me. I was an assistant project manager on a job site. Focusing on work prevented me from dwelling on Jim's situation 24 hours a day. I think that helped me handle all the stress.

Making Decisions

Waiting families may be called upon to make decisions in the course of the patient's treatment. A situation may arise in which so little hope of recovery exists that the family members may be given the option of discontinuing treatment. If this occurs, it is important for all involved in the decision to have very clear information about what has happened to the patient and why the doctors believe that treatment can no longer help. Family members need to discuss what they remember about the patient's opinions about life support when recovery seems unlikely or impossible. Sometimes, the patient has a living will or advanced directive concerning the use of life support in a terminal illness. Many people make such documents because they do not wish to be sustained by machines after meaningful life has ceased. Others, however, leave instructions for all possible measures to be taken. The health care staff will respect the family members' wishes when an ethical choice concerning treatment must be made. It is important for all family members involved in the decision to feel that it is reasonable. Talking things over with a chaplain can often help, even when the medical staff have finished providing all the information they have.

When a person has been declared brain dead, no life support decision has to be made because the person has died, and machinery for life support can automatically be disconnected. However, if the deceased person meets age and other criteria, and has healthy organs and tissues suitable for transplantation into a person whose life can be saved by such a gift, a decision must be made concerning organ donation. Again, the person may have expressed wishes about this in a living will, advance directive, or by signing a donor card or driver's license. Nevertheless, the consent of the legal next-of-kin is required for such a donation, and that person may well prefer to have the agreement of other family members before signing the papers.

At a time of immense distress, often following hours or days of apprehension and suffering, it can be difficult to make a decision that many find controversial. It is a fact, however, that families who agree to donation do not regret it, and that most of them find a unique consolation in the thought of giving hope and new life to others at the time of their own great loss. The opportunity to donate life-giving organs offers a ray of hope in the immense darkness of death. Very few religions discourage such a donation because most generally believe that our earthly bodies decay, return to dust, and cannot be taken to the hereafter. Funerals with open caskets are possible with organ donation because the body is treated with great respect and carefully restored to a condition that permits viewing. In addition to donating vital organs, such as the heart, lungs, kidneys, and liver, it is possible to donate the eyes, parts of which can restore the sight of another person. Again, the donation cannot be detected at the viewing of the body. Families are urged to consider the benefits that organ donation can offer them in their grief. They will be informed of the successful transplantation of the organs. Most report feeling deep consolation as these letters arrive with news of life restored to others.

Asking Spiritual Questions

Regaining spiritual balance may be more helpful than most other remedies for stress. Many people have specific theological questions about the traumatic injury, especially why God allowed it to happen. It is helpful to remember that bad things constantly happen to good people in many different circumstances for no discernible reason. It is also helpful at a time like this to realize that much as human beings desire a just universe in which good is rewarded and evil punished, the reality of the world does not bear this out. Many times good deeds go unrecognized and sometimes bad ones bring their perpetrators rewards; often the innocent die and the guilty live. One reason that the theology of most Christian denominations, and several other religions, nevertheless assert that God is good is that there are values that are constant and transcend life and death and reward and punishment. Christianity names three of these as faith, hope, and love. Christianity, as well as other important world religions, recognizes the existence of suffering and ascribes value and meaning to it. Nowhere does the Bible promise a life free from suffering to any human being, including one who believes in God. It rather asserts that suffering will inevitably occur, that God is present to those who suffer, and that suffering can be transcended.

COMMONLY ASKED QUESTIONS

Why doesn't God perform a miracle?

Miraculous cures have been recorded both in ancient and modern times. But countless prayers for such cures have also been offered without the desired results. Miracles are mysteries, and we do not know why they happen, or when they are going to happen. When people wake from comas that have lasted a long time, it often seems like a miracle. Once people have been declared officially brain dead, according to all scientific criteria, however, they do not wake up.

Recognize that other wonders of God, which do not involve a cure or the undoing of irreversible brain damage, are happening for you. Courage to get through a difficult time, skilled medical staff and others caring for the patient, effective new treatments and medicines, the potential for rehabilitation, and all the love expressed by family members and friends can also be thought of as miracles.

Why do I feel that God has abandoned me?

This is a natural feeling when life has been disrupted and our security has been threatened. In times of great pain and distress people feel alone and abandoned. After the suffering is resolved, a reorientation takes place and we feel connected with others and with life again. Some people are afraid that questioning God's presence or God's will is sinful. It is a natural, spontaneous response to disaster and, if you have ever had a sense of God's presence in your life, you will assuredly find it again. Many who have not yet had this experience will receive it at a time of great need.

Why is God punishing me like this?

We do not know that this is what is happening. Accidents and disasters occur without any discernible reason. If there is a reason, such as a particular human behavior or malicious intent, this reason may not have anything at all to do with God.

Is it sinful to wish that a person die?

This is a natural reaction to extreme injury in another person. The suffering involved in continuing to live after the injury seems unreasonably great and the task of regaining a meaningful life may seem insurmountable. It helps to remember that suffering is not a constant. The injured person's state will change, some improvements and gains may be possible, life goals will be revised, and things that now look hopeless will change and become more hopeful in the future. The task of getting acquainted with and learning to love the person who is injured, with all the changes caused by the injury, may also seem too great to be possible. But, while it is a great task, it can be accomplished little by little over time and, as progress is made, seems much less impossible.

What have we done to deserve this?

The answer is nothing. A brain injury may have been caused by someone's injudicious behavior, but it does not follow that the person injured deserves the terrible consequences.

Beyond these questions, it may eventually be possible to discover new meanings in life, new ways of regarding the self, and new ways of relating to others both for the injured person and for the family. This is an immense spiritual and psychological task that cannot be accomplished overnight. It requires many radical changes in the family system and the way each person approaches life. Change is difficult and slow and may require persistence and patience to make many attempts at the same task. Change always involves grief and suffering for what has been lost, as well as new visions and new rewards. The task of making all these changes is accomplished through the faith, hope, and love that already exist for the family members, and it will create new versions of faith, hope, and love in the lives of all concerned.

CHAPTER 11

The Role of the Social Worker

Amanda L. Hoffmeister, M.S.W., L.C.S.W.

Financial Resources

Patients with head injuries generate costly medical bills and have many needs along the health care continuum. This can be a source of great stress to the patient and family members. The social worker, case manager, or discharge planner can be an excellent resource for navigating through the insurance plan or for applying for resources if the patient does not have insurance. This chapter will discuss insurance coverage and financial resources for head injury patients.

Donna: *The social worker really encouraged me to contact the Social Security office and get things rolling when Sharon was still in the step-down program. I'm glad I did because it takes awhile to get everything going. And oh, I was just so frustrated. I called and said my sister was in a coma and she needed to start Social Security as* *soon as possible because they needed the money. Unbelievably, the woman said, "Well, she needs to call here." I said, "She can't call! She's in a coma!" It was very stressful and aggravating.*

PRIVATE INSURANCE

The patient may be insured through an employer, the spouse's employer, or parents, or may be paying privately for insurance benefits. The best way to define insurance benefits is to refer to the insurance benefit manual. The insurance plan defines deductible amounts, co-pay amounts, and yearly/lifetime maximum amounts. Defining these amounts can assist in planning for future needs. If additional information is needed, the benefits department at the insurance company should be contacted. The social worker can assist with interpretation of the insurance plan and can initiate contact with the insurance company, if requested.

PUBLIC BENEFITS
Medicare

Medicare is a federal health insurance program for people 65 years of age or over. Medicare also provides these benefits to individuals who are under 65 who are considered disabled by Social Security and have received Social Security Disability Income (SSDI) for 24 months. Medicare has benefits for acute hospitalization, acute rehabilitation, skilled rehabilitation, and home health, and pays 80% of some durable medical equipment. All of these benefits must be medically necessary, meet standards as defined by Medicare, and be ordered by a physician. Medicare has two programs, Part A and Part B. Medicare Part A is hospital insurance that pays for inpatient hospital care, skilled nursing care, home health care, and hospice care. Medicare Part A is provided to every individual eligible for Medicare. Medicare Part B helps pay for doctor services, therapies, outpatient services, clinical laboratory services, and home health care. Individuals must pay a monthly premium for Medicare Part B coverage. To obtain a complete description of the Medicare program from the Social Security Administration, the toll-free telephone number is 1-800-772-1213.

Some individuals decide to forfeit their Medicare benefits in exchange for a Medicare HMO plan. A Medicare HMO plan is privatized insurance and is subject to the same conditions previously discussed for private insurance.

Veterans Administration

If the patient served in active military service, he or she may be eligible for benefits through the Veterans Administration. To determine eligibility, contact the Veterans Administration.

State Insurance

Every state has an insurance plan for people who are disabled for a period of time and meet asset requirements. The plans are commonly referred to as "Medicaid," but the name may vary from state to state. The social worker can initiate the application process for Medicaid. These plans typically include benefits for acute inpatient hospitalization, acute rehabilitation, skilled placement, home health care, and medical equipment. All of these benefits must be medically necessary, meet standards as defined by Medicaid, and be ordered by a physician.

Special Children's Programs

Many states offer assistance plans for children or young people injured before the age of 21. The social worker can assist with exploration of these state specific programs.

———❧ COMMONLY ASKED QUESTIONS ❧———

During hospitalization, who communicates the patient's progress and the need for continued hospitalization with the insurance company?

There are typically two ways this information is communicated. A utilization review nurse from the hospital reviews the patient's daily progress and medical treatment and reports this to the insurance company for approval of additional coverage. Or, the insurance company sends a nurse to the hospital to evaluate the patient to certify that continued hospitalization is necessary. If either nurse identifies any concerns about the patient's coverage or need for continued hospitalization, the social worker and physician are notified. The social worker then discusses this with the patient or family members. Many insurance plans refer the patient to an insurance case manager to facilitate this communication.

What is an insurance case manager?

An insurance case manager is usually a nurse or rehabilitation counselor who assists hospital staff in arranging discharge plans within the patient's insurance benefits. Case management can be useful throughout the health care continuum to maximize resources within the patient's insurance plan. The insurance case manager focuses on the organization and sequencing of services and resources specific to the patient.

How does a patient get an insurance case manager?

Often an insurance case manager is a benefit within the patient's insurance plan, especially for catastrophic illnesses. If an insurance case manager is not assigned to the patient, the social worker may request one to assist in discharge planning. The patient should not incur any additional costs for this service and it may help streamline use of the insurance benefits. If a case manager is assigned to the patient, he or she will likely notify the social worker to become involved in planning.

What is "managed care"?

Most insurance companies have formed groups of medical providers (hospitals, physicians, rehabilitation facilities, home health agencies, medical equipment companies, etc.) and are encouraging participants to use services within this group. Common types of managed care are HMOs (Health Maintenance Organizations) and PPOs (Preferred Provider Organizations). If a patient is enrolled in an HMO, all medical care must be coordinated by the patient's primary care physician. A PPO allows the participant a choice of providers within the defined network. PPOs typically do not require referrals from the primary care physician. Other types of managed care insurance plans exist. Refer to the specific insurance plan to define benefits. Medical care provided to patients enrolled in an HMO or PPO is generally classified as either an "in network" or "out of network" service.

What does it mean when a service is "in network" or "out of network"?

"In network" refers to the group of medical service providers with preferred contracts within the insurance plan. Typically, the patient's expense is lower if utilizing these "in network" services. Furthermore, some insurance plans require the use of certain providers for medical care coverage. "Out of network" benefits offer an expanded number of facilities available to participants by allowing the participant to use facilities outside the preferred provider list. Typically, the cost to the patient increases when using an "out of network" facility. Some plans offer no "out of network" benefits. However, if the facility the patient prefers to use is "out of network," the facility may choose to waive the added expenses to the patient to match the patient's "in network" expenses. This is decided on a case-by-case basis and can be explored if the patient is considering an "out of network" provider. If the patient needs to minimize expenses not covered by the insurance plan, it is best to utilize preferred providers. Contact the benefits department of the insurance plan to determine if a facility is "in network."

What options are available if the insurance company denies rehabilitation or other recommended medical services?

If the treatment team strongly recommends rehabilitation or other services, the social worker or physician can advocate for the patient and pursue approval for these services by discussing the patient's needs with the medical director of the insurance plan. The patient may also benefit from family members or employer advocating for the recommended service for the patient. In this circumstance it may be helpful to contact the case manager, provider, employer, or medical director of the insurance plan. The negotiation process for discharge planning requires that the patient has potential for recovery and will benefit from the recommended services. Insurance companies, Medicare, and Medicaid rarely pay for custodial care, or daily, routine care for adult patients. If the patient has no skilled needs at time of discharge, insurance plans will likely not approve these services.

What if the patient does not have health insurance?

The social worker, discharge planner, or case manager will meet with you to discuss your concerns. The options vary, depending on the expected length of disability and the needs of the patient. If the patient meets the financial requirements defined by the state and has a disability, application for the state insurance plan is recommended. If the patient is not anticipated to be disabled for the required time period under the state insurance plan, or if the patient exceeds the financial limits, it may be necessary to complete paperwork informing the hospital of the patient's financial situation. This information is helpful for the hospital to know so that they can make financial plans within the patient's budget.

Does automobile insurance cover medical expenses?

If the patient was injured in a motor vehicle accident, there are certain situations when automobile insurance covers some or all of a patient's medical expenses. However, this can be complicated as the patient's health insurance is typically considered the primary coverage for medical expenses while the automobile insurance coverage is contingent upon liability and settlements. Agreement on insurance coverage from an automobile insurance company can be a very lengthy process. If the patient does not have insurance other than the automobile insurance, the social worker can assist in exploring other resources, such as state insurance programs, to ensure that the patient has coverage for needed services along the health care continuum.

The patient was injured at work; does workers' compensation apply?

If the patient was injured while performing job duties, he or she may be eligible for the employer to cover expenses required to treat the injury. The manager or benefits department at the patient's place of employment has information on workers' compensation benefits.

If the patient formerly had health insurance, could this cover current medical expenses?

Under specific circumstances, the patient may be eligible to continue health insurance coverage. The Consolidated Omnibus Budget Reconciliation Act (COBRA) enables employees to continue group health care coverage from their employer. This act applies to employers with 20 or more employees who provide group health care coverage. There are certain qualifying events that trigger COBRA eligibility, such as the employee's termination of employment, a reduction in hours of employment, divorce or legal separation from a covered spouse, employee's death, or failure to return to work at the end of family and medical leave. Coverage can continue for up to 18, 29, or 36 months depending on the event and situation. If the insured accepts continued insurance coverage through COBRA, he or she is responsible for the full cost of the insurance premium. The employer must notify the insured in writing of the right to continue insurance benefits within 14 days of a qualifying event. To enroll in COBRA insurance benefits, the insured must elect to do so within 60 days after the qualifying event. Talk to the employer's benefits personnel to discuss COBRA insurance questions.

Is financial assistance available for a patient with a brain injury?

The following resources are available to provide monthly income for persons who are disabled for a period of time:

• *Short-term disability from the patient's employer.* If the patient was employed at the time of the hospitalization, the patient may have short-term disability benefits. Not all employers offer this benefit, but if it is available, this benefit provides a percentage of the patient's usual paycheck for a period of time while the patient is disabled. If the patient has this benefit, it is important to determine how long the patient must be considered disabled to receive benefits. Typically, the patient or family members and physician must complete paperwork from the employer.

• *Social Security Disability Income (SSDI).* SSDI provides monthly income for individuals who are expected to be disabled for 1 year or more (or result in death) and who have worked long enough or recently enough for an employer who deducted Social Security withholdings. SSDI has a 6-month waiting period before payments begin from the time that Social Security determines that the patient is disabled. It is important to begin the application process as soon as possible because the process is involved and lengthy. To begin the application process, call 1-800-772-1213. The operator will arrange for either a phone interview or an office visit for you in the future, depending on your preference. Remember to ask the operator what information you will need to gather to be prepared for this interview. Social Security will mail an application and several forms to be signed and returned. The social worker may be able to assist you with these forms. Individuals who have been receiving SSDI for 2 years (24 months) are eligible for Medicare if the disability continues.

• *Supplemental Security Income (SSI).* SSI provides monthly income for individuals who are expected to be disabled for 1 year or more (or result in death) and who have limited assets and income. There is no waiting period for SSI. To begin the application process, call 1-800-772-1213. If the patient is eligible for SSDI, based on work history, and meets the asset limit for SSI, he or she may be eligible for SSI to provide income until the SSDI payments

begin. If the patient is receiving short-term disability from an employer, he or she will not likely be eligible for SSI.

*How can family members manage financial concerns for someone
who is unable to do so?*

Since brain injuries are always unplanned, there often are bills and
financial responsibilities left to be tended to by the family. There
are basically four ways to meet these responsibilities:

1. If the patient completed power of attorney for property prior
to admission, the appointed individual will have access to accounts
and property to care for the patient's financial obligations. Power of
attorney for property is a legal document by which the patient appoints an individual to be responsible for finances and property if
he or she is unable to do so. Immediate family members, personal
lawyers, and the patient's physician may have copies of the power
of attorney.

2. Guardianship is a legal proceeding where a judge appoints an
individual with the responsibility to care for the personal affairs of a
person who has been determined to be incapacitated. The guardian
makes decisions for the incapacitated person within the limits defined by the judge and based on the person's best interests. The
court can also appoint conservatorship to a person that enables that
person to care for financial obligations of the disabled patient.

3. If the patient has another person's name included on the
checking or saving accounts, this person can generally complete financial transactions for the patient.

4. If none of these conditions apply, it is recommended that a
family member contact debtors and notify them in writing of the
hospitalization and general condition of the patient. This docu-
mentation should explain the inability to attend to bills promptly
and request relief from immediate payments to maintain a decent
credit rating.

The financial impact of a brain injury can be overwhelming.
Utilizing resources can be helpful, but it requires patience and per-
severance. Many patients and family members turn to other family
members, churches, and communities to assist with the high costs

of long hospitalizations, the expense of frequent visiting at the hospital or rehabilitation center, and the waiting period until financial assistance begins for the patient.

Choosing a Rehabilitation Facility

As the patient begins to stabilize, the focus shifts from surviving *through* the head injury to living *with* the head injury. This shift in emphasis can raise difficult questions about what to expect in the future, what resources are available, and how the patient accesses these services. One of the team members who will become involved as the patient improves medically is the social worker. The title of this position varies; in some hospitals this person is called the social worker and in others the role is titled "case manager" or "discharge planner." The role of the social worker varies, depending on the patient's needs. You can consult the social worker regarding financial concerns, discharge planning, housing, emotional support, resources, environmental needs like meals and transportation, and choosing the appropriate rehabilitation setting.

One of the greatest fears for family members of patients with a brain injury is that the physician will tell them that the patient will never get better. Often, it is too soon to make these sweeping judgments. You may be wondering if you are able to take the patient home or if there are special resources for recovery or rehabilitation. The social worker will discuss the patient's recovery with the many team members involved in his or her care. The team usually consists of the physician, social worker, nurses, physical, occupational and speech therapists, chaplain, dietitian, and respiratory therapist. As the patient begins to stabilize, the team makes recommendations to meet the patient's needs when he or she is ready to leave the hospital. This decision is based on the patient's progress in therapy, the current neurologic level, the trend of recovery throughout the hospitalization, and the insurance coverage. The social worker then meets with the patient (if he or she is able to participate) and the family members to explore the patient's needs at the time of discharge and the resources available to meet these needs. The final arrangement is called a discharge plan.

The physician determines when the patient is medically stable for discharge. The finalized discharge plan impacts this decision. If the patient is going to a rehabilitation facility, medical conditions can be closely monitored. If the patient is going home or to a skilled nursing facility, the length of hospitalization may be extended to finalize medical treatment. The discharge is canceled if the patient's medical condition changes, requiring continued acute hospitalization.

INPATIENT REHABILITATION

Recovery for patients with head injuries can be very long and slow work. Often, when the physicians, nurses, and social worker begin talking about discharge, the patient is not awake. The goal is to plan for the most appropriate level of rehabilitation; the most common programs are acute, subacute, and skilled. Typically, the social worker discusses the patient's progress with the treatment team to determine the recommended level of rehabilitation. The social worker discusses this recommendation with the family members, makes suggestions for locations, and contacts the facilities to arrange for an evaluation. Often, the rehabilitation facility has an admissions coordinator who will complete an assessment at the hospital. This person can talk to you about the facility, the visiting hours, what clothes or supplies to bring for the patient, and answer specific questions about the facility's program. This person can also arrange a tour of the facility, which can be very helpful in the decision-making process.

> **Sarah:** *I decided which rehabilitation facility Jim should go to. The case worker encouraged us to choose the one affiliated with the hospital . . . and then recommended two other places. . . . I was so impressed I went ahead and enrolled him there. . . . When he was inpatient, I went every day except maybe one.*

Acute Rehabilitation

Acute rehabilitation is the most aggressive level of rehabilitation. Acute rehabilitation is based on the patient tolerating at least 3 hours of therapy everyday. Frequently, the patient must be able to follow commands and show a positive trend in neurologic recovery. Some insurance plans may approve acute rehabilitation while the patient is localizing or making purposeful movements; other plans require a defined level of neurologic function for admission to acute rehabilitation. While in acute rehabilitation the patient works with a team of professionals, including physicians, psychologists, social workers, case manager, nurses, physical therapists, occupational therapists, speech therapists, recreational therapists, and chaplains. One goal of rehabilitation is to encourage the return to routine daily schedules, including sleeping, waking in the morning, getting dressed, and participating in therapy. This can be a challenging adjustment because routine schedules for both the patient and family members have been interrupted during the stressful period in the hospital. The length of time at this level of rehabilitation varies, depending on progress, goals, and insurance coverage.

Acute rehabilitation facilities may be located in hospitals or at independent centers. The visiting hours may be somewhat restricted in this program because the patient will be working very hard and will likely be resting between therapy sessions. This rehabilitation is a crucial step in the recovery process. The options may be limited to a location far from home, especially when looking for a specialized program.

Subacute Rehabilitation

Subacute rehabilitation can be a stepping-stone to acute rehabilitation. This step may extend the amount of time the patient is in rehabilitation, but this level is less costly than acute rehabilitation. Typically, patients have physical, occupational, and speech therapy for up to 3 hours a day. This level of rehabilitation can be beneficial for patients who are making a slow recovery because the amount of therapy is determined by the patient's tolerance. Subacute rehabilitation can be utilized for patients who have medical complications or continue to have significant need for medical care while in rehabilitation.

Specialized Rehabilitation Programs

A specialized facility has nurses, therapists, psychologists, social workers, and physicians who are all specially trained in recovery from a brain injury. These specialized rehabilitation facilities have the specific skills and programs to provide the most aggressive comprehensive rehabilitation available. These programs can apply to receive special accreditation for their program through the Commission on Accreditation of Rehabilitation Facilities (CARF). This organization assesses the program and if it meets the high standards for specialized rehabilitation programs, it can receive CARF accreditation. A facility that receives CARF accreditation for brain injury means that the facility has a special program designed for patients recovering from a brain injury. CARF-accredited programs in general rehabilitation may have a unit for head injuries, so you may want to inquire about the number of individuals served with head injuries and the training of the staff in head injury rehabilitation. If the patient has more than one serious injury, look for a rehabilitation unit that is CARF accredited in more than one area.

Skilled Rehabilitation or Skilled Nursing Facilities

Some patients make slow progress and need time to heal. For patients who are not yet able to tolerate aggressive therapy, the skilled nursing facility offers a skilled environment where the patient can continue to benefit from therapy and have attentive nursing. Not every skilled nursing facility has experience caring for someone with a head injury. The social worker may have a list of those facilities with special programs in a specific area.

It is important to tour these facilities to compare options. When touring, look for cleanliness, patients up and dressed, and an active therapy department with patients receiving therapy. Many times the patient receives minimum therapy at this level of facility. In this case, you may want to meet with the therapists (at the hospital or at the facility) to learn skills to provide range of motion or stimulation therapy to the patient when you are visiting.

GOING HOME

Whether the patient is going home from the rehabilitation facility or from the hospital, this can be an exciting, but also stressful time. Typically, a patient who has suffered a brain injury is physically and/or cognitively different than he or she was before the injury. As such, there are usually changes in the family system that should be addressed prior to discharge home. Some patients require supervision or assistance at home that necessitates altering family member schedules to meet these needs. Preparing for these needs can ease the transition. There are services available for brain injury patients who are ready to be at home but have continued need for assistance or therapy. However, these resources are generally not available for large amounts of time everyday. Prior to discharge, the social worker, case manager, or discharge planner meets with the patient and family members to discuss services necessary for the return home. Recommended services are then arranged by this person.

Hospitalization, rehabilitation, and return home for patients with brain injuries and their families generates incredible stress and anxiety. Knowledge of these resources and options for assistance increases your ability to positively impact the recovery process and enhances your ability to advocate for the patient during this difficult time.

Ellen: *Steve went to outpatient rehabilitation. We brought him straight home from the hospital and he started therapy the following week. We were really lucky. I told him a million times, "Your dad was with you." That's all there was to it. I firmly believe an angel was watching over him.*

Steve had speech therapy and a little bit of physical therapy to get his strength back more than anything. He had lost a tremendous amount of weight and he was a skinny guy anyway. He went from 135 or 140 pounds down to about 115 pounds.

It was scary when I brought him home. I was a little nervous. I was so used to the hospital caring for him. He just wasn't himself and I guess I expected too much. I was being patient but sometimes I was really concerned about his progress. . . . People came over to visit him and said, "Have you gone outside today?" He replied that he had when, of course, he hadn't been outside. It was very odd, but everyday he drifted out a bit in the afternoon. The worst time of the day was about 5 o'clock, when he just kind of went blank. . . . My sister thought that maybe it was because that was the time of the accident. I said, "Oh, my gosh, that's true." However, they don't know enough about the brain to explain the reason.

I was afraid to let him get up and go to the bathroom by himself and I think I drove him crazy. I hovered over him constantly. And, of course, he was a teenager and all he wanted was his privacy! I said, "Steve, I'm your mom, it's okay." But he wanted to take care of himself even while he was still in the hospital. I continued to follow him into the bathroom for awhile and just turned my head! I couldn't let him go alone at first. Finally, I closed the door and sat outside waiting, a nervous wreck!

I think it's important to get away from it, now and then, though. I didn't allow myself time to get away and relax. My husband would suggest that we go somewhere, do something and I would say, "No way." My neighbors came over and suggested we all go out and even offered to stay with Steve, but I said, "No, something will happen while I'm gone." That's just something that's going to be with me the rest of my life . . . the constant worry, it's constant.

❦ COMMONLY ASKED QUESTIONS ❦

How will the transfer occur?

When the physician determines the patient is medically stable for discharge and the discharge plan has been finalized, the social worker arranges appropriate transportation. Many patients are transported by ambulance to the rehabilitation or nursing facility. If the patient is being transported by ambulance, one person may be able to ride with the patient. Although this is not required, it may be supportive to the patient.

Will my insurance pay for rehabilitation?

Private, federal, and state insurance plans generally provide benefits for rehabilitation. All have specific requirements for eligibility. The impact of insurance has been discussed earlier in this chapter.

When is a patient ready for discharge from inpatient rehabilitation?

During rehabilitation, there should be meetings where all of the members of the rehabilitation team, the patient, and family members address the patient's progress toward rehabilitation goals. These goals are based on the patient's home environment, insurance coverage, and expectation for recovery. During these meetings, a schedule will be developed for the patient's discharge from the rehabilitation facility. As the patient's discharge date approaches, the rehabilitation team, patient, and family members will determine whether the patient should proceed to a skilled nursing facility, a residential/supportive living program, a state-sponsored acute rehabilitation center, or home.

What is a residential/supportive living program?

A residential/supportive living program focuses on social reintegration through activities of daily living, self-help skills, socialization, and counseling. The object is to restore the patient to the optimal level of physical, cognitive, and behavioral functioning. These programs are generally facilitated by nurses, therapists, and social workers. These programs may be available on either an inpatient or outpatient basis.

What is a state-sponsored acute rehabilitation program?

State rehabilitation facilities can provide extended acute rehabilitation, depending on the patient's insurance coverage. Check with your rehabilitation social worker to determine if your state has a state-sponsored acute rehabilitation facility and the eligibility requirements for this program.

What is a skilled nursing facility, nursing home, or long-term care facility?

This type of facility provides a skilled environment to meet the needs of a patient whose physical care exceeds the capabilities of family members.

What are the services available for the patient who can be discharged home, but has continued need for treatment?

The options for care at this point are home health care, outpatient therapy, day treatment, and vocational rehabilitation. Home health services include physical therapy, occupational therapy, speech therapy, social work, psychiatric nursing, nurses aides, and registered nurses who visit home-bound patients at their residence. A physician's order is needed to arrange home health care. As discussed previously, the social worker, case manager, or discharge planner will arrange recommended services prior to discharge.

Outpatient therapy is continued through scheduled appointments at a local therapy center. These centers are either independent therapy businesses or therapy departments at hospitals. A physician must write a prescription for these services and the patient must present this prescription to the therapy center.

Day treatment is an intensive outpatient therapy program. This program is most helpful when multiple therapies are needed. Day treatment programs are often associated with rehabilitation facilities offering specialized brain injury rehabilitation. The social worker, case manager, or discharge planner will arrange day treatment prior to discharge.

Vocational rehabilitation is a program that addresses the necessary skills and education to return to work or learn new job skills. The name and specifics of this program vary by state. This service can be provided in conjunction with home health care, outpatient, or day treatment. The social worker, case manager, or discharge planner may initiate this service for the patient.

Are there specific resources for emotional support and information for family members of patients with head injuries?

Often there are support groups for family members of brain injury patients. Check with your social worker for information about the support groups offered in your area. Additionally, many states have a brain injury association that maintains a list of support groups throughout the state. Aside from support groups, a brain injury association can provide information on medical advancements, legal issues, and available counseling, and publishes a quarterly newsletter that includes much of this information. You may choose to become involved with the local chapter to advocate for the needs of people surviving with a head injury, to stay up to date on head injury resources and information, or to meet others with similar experiences. The Internet may be another resource to research information on brain injuries.

Where should the patient turn for help with legal issues?

It is best to consult an attorney for specific legal concerns. Attorneys may specialize in automobile insurance settlements, workers' compensation claims, Social Security disability appeals, guardianship, or other areas of specific concerns. If finances limit the options for attorneys, the social worker can provide information on local resources for low-cost legal assistance.

PART

II

THE NEXT STEP

REHABILITATION

CHAPTER
12

❦

Aspects of Therapy

Christopher Kuseliauskas, R.N.

The rehabilitation process begins as soon as the patient has been medically stabilized. The first step is to assess the patient to determine the level of dysfunction. Once the patient is evaluated, appropriate rehabilitation professionals are incorporated into the existing health care team. This process may begin when the patient is still in the **intensive care unit** or **ICU,** but long-term rehabilitation needs are typically determined after the patient has been moved out of the ICU and into a floor bed.

The main goal of rehabilitation is to help the patients and family members return to their previous level of functioning. The amount and type of rehabilitative efforts depend on the amount of brain damage and the resultant functional loss sustained by the patient. If the patient has suffered a major brain injury, extensive inpatient and outpatient rehabilitation are usually necessary. Patients with mild to moderate injury may require less therapy, focused on specific needs, such as cognitive issues or vocational retraining.

As the rehabilitation evaluation process begins, the long-term consequences of the head injury become apparent. A loved one has survived a very traumatic experience and the attention now shifts from life-and-death issues to attempts at making a functional recovery. Most acute medical issues have been resolved and postinjury issues, such as cognitive, behavioral, memory, language, and mobility problems, take center stage. The transition from the acute hospital setting to the rehabilitation setting can be a time of stress, not only because patients and family members must learn new names, faces, and routines, but the entire dynamics of the family may be disrupted, as members of the family are forced to take on new responsibilities, roles, and duties.

REHABILITATION LEVELS AND THEIR ADMISSION CRITERIA

The amount and type of rehabilitation are based entirely on the patient's needs. These are typically determined by rehabilitation specialists during the acute medical phase. The patient is assessed by a physical therapist or PT, occupational therapist or OTR, and a speech therapist or SPT. Following this assessment they recommend what services are needed. Patients with minor injuries and little or no functional deficits may not require any rehabilitation, while others with severe injury may require long-term, aggressive services. Again, it should be kept in mind that, in general, the amount of damage sustained to the brain roughly correlates with the amount of rehabilitation necessary. Depending on the functional deficits, the rehabilitation specialists will recommend whether the patient needs to go to an acute inpatient rehabilitation center, inpatient subacute center, or an outpatient facility. It is important that wherever the patient goes for rehabilitation the facility be accredited and specialize in neurologic dysfunction.

Acute inpatient rehabilitation is the most aggressive. This type is usually associated with a major medical facility and may be part of a hospital complex or freestanding (separate, in its own building). These facilities have specialized services to deal with different types of rehabilitation needs, including neurorehabilitation. It is staffed like an acute hospital and can handle most medical issues that may arise during rehabilitation.

Most acute rehabilitation facilities provide therapy utilizing a multidisciplinary approach, meaning that each patient is assigned a team, which includes the patient and family members. The team also includes a medical director, nurses, physical therapists, occupational therapists, speech therapists, and a social worker. The focus is individual treatment based on the patient's needs.

> **Sarah:** *I visited Jim everyday in rehabilitation. I think it was important that I went, although during the therapy they discourage interruptions and distractions. So I worked, went home, got the kids settled, and then went to see him in the evenings. Finally, they wanted me to come see him at one of his therapy sessions. That was nice because I could see how he was progressing. I could tell he was real emotional. He knew he was still having trouble with some things and that was hard. He felt helpless, and that was hard for a man like Jim.*
>
> *They had him playing ball, throwing it back and forth. Seemingly simple physical things. Then they asked him questions. Once he blurted out, "I can't even remember the f*?#$@! alphabet." He was really distressed; he cried a lot.*
>
> *It was important to remember the patient's ego—his feelings—not to try and do everything for him, but to let him show me how he was progressing and be supportive."*

The admission criteria for acute, inpatient rehabilitation are that the patient must be able to tolerate 3 hours of therapy a day and be medically stable. Patients considered medically stable are those who do not have any ongoing, unresolved, acute medical issues, such as fever, ventilator requirements, or cardiovascular instability. Hence, not all head injury patients are candidates for acute inpatient rehabilitation. Although the ability to tolerate 3 hours of therapy a day does not sound like much, it may initially be quite a challenge for a severe head injury patient. Obviously, patients who remain unconscious are not able to undergo intensive therapy and thus are not candidates for this type of rehabilitation until their condition improves.

Another requirement for an acute inpatient admission is that the patient must require services from at least two of the three different rehabilitation disciplines (physical, occupational, and speech therapy). For instance, patients with no medical issues and who only require PT for an unsteady gait may be able to receive rehabilitation in a less intensive subacute setting or as an outpatient.

The range of patients who can be admitted to an acute inpatient setting can vary widely. All the various factors, both medical and rehabilitative, are weighed together to ascertain whether a patient should be admitted to an acute inpatient facility or whether some other type of facility would be better suited to address the patient's needs.

Subacute inpatient rehabilitation may be more appropriate for a patient who cannot meet the acute rehabilitation requirements because of an inability to tolerate the intensive therapy or, for whatever reason, does not require the extensive services provided by acute rehabilitation. Subacute rehabilitation is a good option for the patient who needs to build up endurance to prepare for the more intense acute rehabilitation. Many patients who are still comatose or functioning at a very low neurologic level start their rehabilitation here and, as they progress, are transferred to an acute facility. Patients who were admitted to the acute rehabilitation and who may be having some difficulty tolerating the intensity may find subacute rehabilitation helpful in building up their endurance and tolerance. Many acute rehabilitation facilities have subacute beds just for these purposes.

The subacute units have all the services of the more acute units, including physicians, nurses, occupation, physical, and speech therapists. They also utilize the multidisciplinary approach. Sometimes family members view placement in a subacute center as a step backward, but it is important to remember that it is best to match the level of rehabilitation with the patient's ability to make the efforts most effective.

Long-term rehabilitation is indicated for those who have survived severe injuries and have completed the acute inpatient rehabilitation but need continued therapy without extensive medical monitoring. The focus is the same as acute rehabilitation, that being functional recovery, but it has a longer term focus that may last months or years and may include a residential treatment component to help the patient return to the community.

Outpatient rehabilitation usually involves the patient going home and then either going to a facility for rehabilitation or receiving rehabilitation in the home. Again, the amount and intensity depend on the patient's needs. Patients at home may still require nurses to make home visits to administer medications or wound care. Many begin outpatient therapy following discharge from the acute inpatient rehabilitation facility. The focus and goal of outpatient rehabilitation is basically a continuation of the progress that the patient had made during the more aggressive therapies. This is also the point at which the patient may begin to focus on returning to work, running a household, or going back to school.

GOALS OF REHABILITATION

It would be difficult within the scope of this chapter to discuss all the various prognosis issues and potential rehabilitation needs for every different head injury patient. Every brain injury is a unique event and no two patients are the same. Age is not necessarily a good prognostic determinate in terms of functional impairment, given that a young and old brain are *both* composed of the tissue (neurons) that does not regenerate once damaged. Although younger people tend to survive trauma more often than older patients, the long-term consequences of head injury and, hence, the amount of rehabilitation needed, are generally based on the severity of the brain injury. The more the brain has been damaged, the greater the need for long postacute care.

COGNITIVE DYSFUNCTION

The two general categories addressed by head injury rehabilitation are cognitive and physical dysfunctions. **Cognition** refers to the thinking, personality, behavior, memory, speech, and language skills. Cognition also involves how we interpret and process information from our environment and how we react and respond to that information. The **frontal lobes** of the brain are the main centers for cognitive control, while the **temporal lobes** are the main sites for memory. Unfortunately, these two areas are usually the most affected after a brain injury. Even a mild injury may cause some cognitive dysfunction and memory loss. Speech and language problems (including **aphasia**) can occur when there is damage to the dominant (usually the left) hemisphere.

> **Donna:** *I asked about Sharon's memory. The doctor explained that her injury was all over the brain, not confined to one spot. The brain was bruised everywhere, which was why they never could tell us, "She might have trouble remembering this or that." They always said, "We don't know." When she was still in the coma, we always entered her room with "Hi, Sharon, it's November 16th and it's rainy or snowy or whatever. This is Donna, I'm your sister." We hoped that this would help her later when she tried to remember everything.*
>
> *She has no memories of the day of the accident. Her memory is very selective, although some of her cognitive abilities returned right away. When she started to talk, we were constantly taking her down the hall in the wheelchair. She wanted to be on the move constantly, not just stay in that room. As we passed different doors, she read the signs on them, like "mechanical room." She could read that and everything else. We were amazed that she could read, after all she had been through. She may not have been able to even say who you were at that time, but she could read. That was very reassuring.*

The Rancho Los Amigos scale is an assessment tool used by many rehabilitation professionals to help categorize a patient's cognitive functioning. The scale divides cognitive ability into eight different levels.

• **Level I: No Response.** The patient is unresponsive to any stimuli. This means that the patient does not respond to a person's voice, touch, or even pain. This level includes those patients who are deeply unconscious (in a coma). Rehabilitation goals in this situation are to consistently introduce various forms of stimuli in an attempt to solicit a response. This is commonly referred to as "coma stimulation."

• **Level II: Generalized Response.** The patient reacts inconsistently and nonpurposely to stimuli. These responses may be physiologic changes, such as changes in the blood pressure or heart rate in response to a voice or touch, gross body movements, or vocalizations. These reactions to stimuli may also be very delayed. Some specialists have also categorized this level as a comatose state.

Rehabilitation goals include consistent, structured therapy sessions with the goal to have the patient demonstrate more consistent responses and follow very simple, one-step commands.

• **Level III: Localized Response.** Responses are directly related to the type of stimulus presented, but still may be inconsistent. These patients may follow simple commands in an inconsistent delayed manner. In some instances, certain patients may respond to some individuals better than others.

It usually takes the parents or loved ones of the patient some time to convince the rehabilitation staff that the patient is at this level. This is one reason why family members are so important during the rehabilitation process. Patients usually do more for some one they know or are comfortable with. The patient may also have a favorite therapist or staff member, and consistently does more for those individuals. The rehabilitation goals again include looking for more consistent responses and command following.

• **Level IV: Confused and Agitated.** These patients are in a heightened state of activity with severely decreased ability to process information. Behavior is frequently bizarre and nonpurposeful relative to the environment. Gross attention is often very short and selective attention is virtually nonexistent.

At this level the patient reacts to any stimulus in the environment and can easily become agitated. The goal is to provide the patient with a structured, low-stimulation environment. This involves putting the patient on a schedule and, at times, limiting the amount of visitors. Various stimuli are introduced in short sessions, allowing time for the patient to process the information and respond. It is at this stage that the therapist begins to work one-on-

one with the patient, in a quiet environment. This helps to decrease outside, unwanted stimuli and allows the patient to focus on the therapist. Initially, the patient may be highly distractible, with the resultant attention span being so short that focus on a particular rehabilitation task can only be kept for a few seconds.

The patient also requires a strict, 24-hour supervision. Family members may be asked to assist with this. A Vail Bed or similar device may also be recommended. These special beds allow the patient to move about freely in bed without restraints, but they have special netting to prevent patients from falling out of the bed or injuring themselves.

• **Level V: Confused, Inappropriate, Non-Agitated.** The patient appears alert and is able to consistently follow simple commands, but continues to be highly distractible and lacks the ability to focus attention on specific tasks for long periods of time. Memory can be severely impaired, leading to confusion for the past and present. These patients typically have a difficult time learning new information.

> **Sarah:** *Jim had problems with reading, with focusing and concentrating. He kept saying his eyes needed to be checked or asked me to get him reading glasses. But it really wasn't his eyes, it was his brain. It was hard to explain that to him. He used to read quite a bit and then suddenly he didn't understand. Now he is reading pretty well again.*

At this stage the patient is, however, able to tolerate longer therapy sessions, although the environment must still be highly structured and "low-stimulation" because the patient continues to lack insight and problem-solving skills. Combined with memory difficulties, it is difficult for the patient to learn and retain new skills. Therapy therefore focuses on tasks that are repetitious and require less reasoning and abstract thinking skills.

The patient is typically less agitated at this time and may begin to participate in more group activities, but often require redirection to stay on task. Inappropriate behaviors can still occur and social skills are usually nonexistent, with the patient having a difficult time controlling inhibitions. This difficulty can manifest as sexually inappropriate actions or the use of harsh language.

• **Level VI: Confused, Appropriate.** The patient shows goal directed behavior and begins to follow more complex commands. Responses may be inaccurate due to memory problems, but are generally more appropriate to the situation, resulting in the ability to carry out functional activities. These patients are consistently oriented to person, time, and place (i.e., they know who they are, where they are, and what time or season it is).

At this point the patient is able to perform more complex rehabilitation tasks and tolerate longer rehabilitation sessions. The patient begins to participate in self-care skills, such as toileting, grooming, and feeding. Behavioral issues are generally less of a concern at this level, but insight, processing, and problem-solving skills continue to be limited.

• **Level VII: Automatic, Appropriate.** The patient is appropriate and oriented within familiar settings and is able to complete daily routines, although it may be in a robot-like manner. There may be some awareness of the condition, but insight is typically lacking. Poor judgment and problem-solving skills continue.

This may be the point at which some patients leave the inpatient rehabilitation setting and begin outpatient or long-term rehabilitation. These patients do well in a structured, familiar environment, like the hospital or home, but have a difficult time in unfamiliar settings, such as the grocery store, at work, or at school.

• **Level VIII: Purposeful, Appropriate.** The patient is alert and oriented and able to integrate past and recent events. He or she requires no supervision once the task has been learned and is independent in home and community activities. Challenges may be noted in abstract reasoning, tolerance for stress, or judgment in stressful situations.

These patients usually only require a short inpatient rehabilitation stay or may go directly into an outpatient program. Goals here are to evaluate the patient's ability to return to a vocational or school setting.

Ellen: *Steve had a lot of short-term memory loss in the beginning, but even as sick as he was and with so much pain, his sense of humor never left him. Once, during rehabilitation the speech therapist working with him and I came into the room. She asked him who I was. He replied, "I don't know." Well, I just about lost it. I was afraid he was having a terrible setback. I thought, "Oh, my God." I got a little bit closer and I said, "Steve, you know who I am." Again he said, "No." Tears rolled down my face and I asked him again, "Who am I?" He said, "I know who you are, Mom, I'm just giving you a hard time!" The little pistol! When he pulled that stunt I knew he was going to be fine, he was going to be just fine.*

The levels mentioned above are only a guide to help determine a patient's cognitive function. While these levels are helpful in evaluating patients, they have no predictive value. A patient who starts out at a very low level may show little to no progression despite intensive therapy. There is never a guarantee a patient will improve. Some may remain at a particular level indefinitely. Patients who have sustained a moderate to severe head injury will most likely experience long-term problems with regard to cognitive function and may require long-term rehabilitation or vocational training. The important point to remember is that recovery from significant brain injury is often a long, arduous process.

Physical Dysfunctions

In addition to cognitive deficits, head injury patients may also have a certain degree of physical dysfunction. The type and severity of these physical impairments depends on *both* the area and the extent of the brain damage. As with cognitive dysfunction, the more extensive the brain injury, typically the more extensive the physical disability.

The physical symptoms that affect mobility and self-care issues are very similar to the symptoms that occur after a stroke. For example, a stroke that occurs on the left side of the brain results in weakness on the right side of the body. In both stroke and head injuries, the more the brain is adversely affected, the greater the amount of weakness. The frontal lobe is the location of the **motor area** (i.e., the area that controls movement in the body) and is, in part, responsible for muscle strength. Weakness on one side of the body is referred to as **hemiparesis.** This is usually graded on a scale of 1 to 5, with 1 being the weakest and 5 being normal strength. Complete paralysis on one side of the body is termed **hemiplegia.** Rarely is there complete weakness or paralysis that affects *both* upper or *both* lower extremities, unless there is an associated spinal cord injury or extensive damage to *both* hemispheres of the brain. The muscles that control swallowing can also become weak, causing **dysphagia** (difficulty swallowing). When the muscles that help us with speech become weak, the words sound slurred, which is called **dysarthria.**

Muscle tone of the affected or weak extremities is also a concern after a brain injury. Tone refers to how relaxed or contracted an arm or leg is when the extremity is at rest. The tone in the affected arm or leg (or both) can range from "flaccid" (i.e., completely limp) to a state of "hypertonicity," meaning the extremity is constantly contracted and tight. Increased tone can cause problems with range of motion and eventually lead to **contractures** (i.e., permanent fixation of the limb in a particular position).

Apraxia may also be present after the injury. This term means that the patient has difficulty utilizing the extremity during a functional task, such as getting dressed. The problem is not due to weakness but rather due to an inability by the brain to produce adequate motor *planning* for the task, for example, a patient who is asked to brush the hair with a comb, but instead attempts to brush the teeth. The patient may be able to complete the task spontaneously, but associated cognitive problems make it difficult to complete the task on command.

Balance and coordination problems may also exist after injury, especially if the **cerebellum** has been affected. This is known as **ataxia** (i.e., problem with stability) and may cause problems with mobility or performing self-care skills, such as walking or standing in a shower.

Sarah: Balance was a problem for Jim at first. Once he was in rehabilitation, they worked on that with physical therapy, not only to get his strength back but also to improve his balance. Whenever he was on uneven ground, he fell or tripped. But he's fine now and his balance has returned to normal.

Patients with physical impairments may also lack the necessary endurance to fully participate in PT and OT. Patients who had complicated medical courses and spent a large amount of time in the ICU especially need time to build up their endurance. Learning to ambulate again or trying to compensate for a weak side takes an enormous amount of endurance. Initially, even patients who sustain a mild injury may have problems with endurance and fatigue.

Sensory and visual problems, which may be present after a brain injury, can also compound the picture and make it difficult for the patient to appropriately utilize the arms and/or legs in certain activities. These are known as "perceptual motor skills." These can manifest as difficulties with positional sense of an arm or leg or knowing the position or location of a body part in space. A decreased ability to feel touch can leave the affected extremity feeling numb, making certain movements awkward. For example, patients who cannot feel their feet have a difficult time walking because they cannot feel their feet on the ground. Vision problems, such as peripheral visual loss or visual field deficits, can produce **hemianopsia** or different types of **quadranopsia** (i.e., superior, inferior). Blurred or double vision can also occur. Patients with these abnormalities may have difficulty turning corners or reacting to visual objects within their environment.

The combination of hemiparesis, loss of sensation on one side, and hemianopsia can lead to a syndrome called **neglect.** Loosely translated, this means that the patient tends to ignore the world on the affected side. This can make tasks such as self-care, bathing, eating, and ambulating quite difficult and cause some potential safety issues. These patients need to possess a high level of insight and awareness to compensate for the neglect.

THE MULTIDISCIPLINARY
REHABILITATIVE TEAM

The multidisciplinary team is a highly dynamic unit. The goals for the patient are never static and change according to the patient's needs. As the patient progresses, additional and more challenging goals are introduced. It is important to remember that no one discipline has any more importance than the other. The team, made up of the medical director, registered nurses, and physical, occupational, speech, and recreational therapists, collectively works together to help the patient and family achieve their goals.

The medical director (MD) oversees the medical care for the patient and typically has specialized training in rehabilitation. The medical director ensures that the patient remains medically stable and monitors any potential medical problems. Most acute, inpatient rehabilitation centers can handle the majority of medical issues, but if more serious problems occur, the medical director may consult other professionals.

Registered nurses (RNs) work closely with the MDs, to help monitor the patient's medical status and medications, and with the therapy staff, especially when the patient still requires close medical observation during therapy sessions. They spend a great deal of time educating the patient and family members about medications, as well as medical and nursing issues.

The social worker (SW) usually holds a master's degree and works closely with family members with regard to community, state, and federal resources available. They also meet with the patient and family members to help determine what their rehabilitation goals are. At discharge, the social worker plays a significant role in ensuring that all plans are in place and that all equipment or resources have been obtained. The social worker also helps the family find long-term rehabilitation placement or facility and coordinates home health services if needed. They spend a great deal of time educating the family and providing support.

Registered occupational therapists (OTs) are rehabilitation professionals who have completed a master's degree. They may supervise a certified occupational therapy assistant (COTA). OTs help the patient regain self-care skills, including dressing, bathing, grooming, and eating. As such, the OTs focus on skills that require use of the upper extremities and evaluate the patient's range of motion, strength, and tone. If a high level of tone is present, the OT may utilize serial casting or splinting techniques to help decrease the tone. Cognitively, OTs focus on skills such as attention, concentration, organization, problem solving, insight, safety awareness, and memory. OTs evaluate the patient's need for any assistive devices that may be necessary to increase the patient's ability to complete self-care skills. They also work with patients who demonstrate poor perceptual motor skills, such as neglect or apraxia, and help patients compensate for any visual difficulties that may be present. OTs work with patients both individually and in group settings, if the patient can participate.

Registered physical therapists (PTs) usually hold a bachelor's or master's degree. They may supervise a physical therapy assistant (PTA), who has an associate degree. A PT's main focus is mobility and lower extremity issues. For mild injuries, PTs may only address high-level balance or safety issues. For severe injuries, they may initially work on increasing endurance, as well as work with the patient on tolerating a more upright position, given that most of these patients have spent the majority of time in bed. They incorporate cognitive skills, such as insight, awareness, navigational skills, and problem solving, into their therapy sessions. They are also responsible for evaluating the patient and ordering any necessary adaptive equipment (i.e., wheelchairs, canes, or other ambulation aids). They closely evaluate the patient's range of motion and strength and monitor for increased tone or spasticity. Like all the therapy disciplines, PTs work with patients both in individual and group sessions.

Speech therapists (SPTs) are also educated at the master's level. They assess the patient's speech and language abilities, including oral, written, and nonverbal communication, to evaluate for the presence of aphasia or dysarthria. They also complete a thorough cognitive evaluation and develop a treatment plan consistent with the patient's level of functioning. They evaluate the patient's ability to swallow to detect dysphagia. If the patient has a G-tube in place, the SPT routinely evaluates the patient's oral structures and determines when the patient may be ready to begin taking in oral food.

> **Donna:** *Sharon's speech is still not like it was, of course, but she's getting a lot better. I said, "Sharon, when you read a book, read out loud. It will improve your speech. The more you talk, the more you read out loud, it will make things better.*
>
> *She passed her swallow test before leaving the rehabilitation center and could have very soft foods but nothing more "watery" than a "honey-like" consistency so she didn't choke. . . . For instance, she could eat a scrambled egg but she could not drink water, or lemonade, or coffee. She couldn't have anything like that. Everything liquidy had to be thickened. Soup had to be thickened.*

SPTs also work with patients who have tracheostomy tubes in place to improve their communication skills and, if indicated, help patients prepare to have the tracheotomy removed. This is accomplished by plugging the tracheotomy for periods of time until the patient is able to tolerate it being plugged for longer than 24 hours. SPTs work in conjunction with the medical and respiratory therapy staff to safely accomplish this.

Recreational therapists (RTs) are professionals focused on incorporating all the learned rehabilitation skills into social and community environments. RTs may take patients on "out trips" into the community. This allows the patient to transfer skills learned in the hospital into real-world situations. For example, taking patients to a grocery store allows them to practice skills such as mobility, problem solving, and communication. These out trips give the therapist excellent feedback on how the patient can handle these situations and may help in developing a relevant care plan. The recreational therapist also develops group sessions that may include games that test memory and attention skills or crafts that help with problem-solving skills and the use of the upper extremities.

The program and assistant program directors usually have a background in rehabilitation and many were former OTs, PTs, or SPTs. They ensure that their particular program is running smoothly and that all the patient's needs are being met. They also ensure that a care plan has been developed that is appropriate for the individual patient's needs. They also typically run weekly meetings that include the entire rehabilitation team, including the patient and family members. It is at these meetings that the team discusses how the patient is doing with regard to attaining goals and if new, more challenging ones need to be added. If the patient is having difficulty attaining the goals, it may be necessary for the goals to be changed. It is the program director who communicates this information to the insurance companies and case managers. Some case managers may even be present at these meetings. It is important that the patient show progress and that the goals are attainable. If not, the insurance company may hesitate at providing funding for services.

Other professionals that patients and family members may encounter include respiratory therapists and registered dietitians. If the patient still requires a tracheotomy for airway protection, the respiratory therapist ensures that there are no problems and assists the medical team and SPT when attempting to "wean" the patient from the trach (i.e., slowly withdraw and eventually remove the tracheostomy tube).

The registered dietitian ensures that the patient is using the correct diet. Caloric needs after a brain injury are quite high and the dietitian monitors each patient to ensure that the patient is receiving adequate intake related to increased needs. They also work with the SPT on patients who have swallowing difficulties and educate the patient and family members regarding any special diets or tube feedings, if indicated.

Sarah: Jim said his first words on day 19. He said, "You bet." Then on the day 20 he ate by himself. They finally gave him real food. Most people have trouble swallowing after a head injury. Tubes have been placed in their throats and the muscles forget how to work. That was a big milestone. It was really strange because before that, when I brought Hanna, our baby, to the hospital, he took her juice bottle out of my hand, unscrewed the cap, and drank it! He hadn't been given anything by mouth up until then. He remembers doing that. He said he was thirsty!

—❧ COMMONLY ASKED QUESTIONS ❧—

How does the process of discharge from the hospital to rehabilitation facility work?

Once the patient's rehabilitation needs have been determined by the hospital rehabilitation staff, the social worker begins to coordinate the transfer to the appropriate center after the patient is medically cleared by the health care team. This is done in conjunction with the family members, who are provided options on what facilities are available in the area. The social worker also addresses relevant insurance issues. In those instances where the patient has no insurance, the social worker helps to determine what type of state and/or federal aid may be available. After a facility has been chosen, a representative confirms the patient's needs and most appropriate level of rehabilitation. This individual is usually a registered nurse who specializes in rehabilitation, but nonmedical individuals with rehabilitation experience may also be involved. These representatives should provide the patient and family members with a thorough description of the facility and the services offered. In some instances, several different rehabilitation centers may be available. It is highly advisable to tour the prospective facility and have any and all questions answered at that time. When deciding on a particular rehabilitation facility, be sure that it is CARF accredited. This means that the facility has been evaluated by an independent agency and found to meet the minimum standards in providing rehabilitation.

> **Donna:** *We all talked very openly and shared in the decision making about Sharon's care. None of the facilities was near our home, so we were still going to be doing a lot of commuting. The social worker provided us with information about various centers, and we asked the family members of other patients for their recommendations. One mother whose son was in an accident and was doing really well in rehabilitation said such wonderful things about the facility they had chosen, we selected the same center for Sharon.*
>
> *It is also important to talk to the nurses. Some said, "Well, you didn't hear this from me, but you definitely don't want to go there. I took their advice and listened to the other patient's family members. We were all there the day Sharon was moved to the rehabilitation center.*

Prior to discharge to the rehabilitation site, the therapists who had been working with the patient in the hospital typically educate the family members as to the current types of dysfunction the patient may be experiencing. This information will be very useful in the acute rehabilitation stage because the family becomes a big part of the rehabilitative team. Take this opportunity to learn as much as you can, because chances are, you will eventually become the most important therapist for your loved one.

What about prognosis or recovery after a head injury?

When we discuss long-term prognosis, we are referring to what the patient and family members might encounter in the next 6 months to years after surviving a head injury. We can only try to answer this question in a general manner, since as stated earlier, no two injuries are the same. Prognosis depends on many factors, with the most significant being the extent of the primary and secondary brain damage. The general rule is, the more of the brain that was damaged, the more severe the long-term consequences and care needed. The important thing to remember is that recovery from a brain injury takes a long time. Recovery is not measured in days or weeks, but in months and years. Another important point to remember is that, initially, progress and recovery may be quite rapid, but then slows down or may even plateau. The recovery process can also follow a peak and valley scenario, where progress occurs at irregular intervals. No two patients follow the same path. Setbacks are more common than not, especially if the patient has concurrent medical problems during rehabilitation. Progress can also slow down if the patient is experiencing fatigue, has not been eating, or is having trouble sleeping. Depression is also common after a head injury and, at times, the patient may want to give up or not participate in therapies. These same problems can occur after the patient has completed rehabilitation. It is important for the family members to learn as much as possible about the mechanism of brain injury so they fully understand what hurdles and challenges their loved one is facing. This allows the family members to be fully integrated into the rehabilitation team and to become advocates for the survivor in the long term.

Donna: *The holidays were approaching so we had decorations in Sharon's room and cards everywhere. The nurses said not to overdo because that's not good for her either. We just put up a certain amount of cards and then changed them every so often.*

When her son's birthday was coming up, we tried to get her excited. We told her, "Sharon, Brian's birthday is coming" and we looked hard to see some response. I always liked to think she actually heard me. Looking back on it, sometimes I think I just looked too hard. Maybe she did open her eyes, but she might have opened them anyway, as a reflex.

I didn't want to show any negative feelings. I didn't want to cry in front of her. Sometimes I did and I just tried to hurry up and get myself back in control. And we didn't talk about any negative things in front of her, only positive. We told her what was going on, "Brian is on the wrestling team and you know he won his match"; anything and everything good about the family.

She doesn't have any bitterness, but she's depressed. She wants her life back. That's what she says a lot, "I want my life back and it's just taking so long. I never thought it would take this long." She doesn't remember certain things. She doesn't remember that our mother passed away in 1991 and our grandmother passed away in 1990. She also doesn't remember either of our grandpas, both of whom passed away in the 1970s. She doesn't remember her wedding day. She doesn't remember giving birth to her children, she doesn't remember any of this. But she can remember her girlfriend from high school who came to see her in the hospital. She remembers her friends, she remembers all of us, and she can tell me how to get somewhere, driving.

When she came home, was it a really big day or was it sort of subdued? It was not a big celebration. Sharon was so sick of the hospital, sick of the nurses. She just couldn't stand it any longer. Toward the end of her hospitalization, she constantly yelled, "Nurse, Nurse," which I know was very irritating for the nurses because it was irritating for me! I said, "Sharon, quit calling for the nurse. She can't do anything. Everything's okay, I'm here with you and we'll go for a walk, we'll get out of here." She kept saying, "I feel like I'm having a breakdown." Of course, she wasn't speaking clearly and it was very hard to understand her. She's come a long way with her speech, but at first I couldn't even understand basic words.

Individuals who have sustained a mild head injury have the best chance of recovery and returning to an independent lifestyle. Mild head injury usually means that the patient's **Glasgow Coma Scale** at the time of the accident was quite high, with little or no loss of consciousness at the scene and a fairly uncomplicated acute hospital stay. The most common problems encountered after a mild injury usually involve problems with cognitive skills, including lack of attention to detail, distractibility, mental fatigue, problem-solving and insight skills, skills that require divided attention, and a lower frustration or stress tolerance. Utilizing the Ranchos Los Amigos scale, the mild head injury survivor functions at the higher levels. However, the patient may demonstrate some short-term or recent memory difficulties. From a mobility standpoint, the patient may demonstrate problems in the areas of high-level balance skills, decreased endurance, and fatigability, or upper and/or lower extremity weakness. These difficulties may become significantly better over time, but even the mild head injury survivor may have long-term problems with any one or a combination of these issues.

These patients may require a short acute inpatient rehabilitation stay, but will probably spend the majority of the time in an outpatient setting with the goal of returning to work, school, or home.

On the other end of the spectrum is the survivor of a severe head injury. Severe means an individual who has sustained extensive primary and secondary brain damage and had a very low Glasgow Coma Scale score during the first 24 to 48 hours after the injury. These patients require aggressive medical intervention and usually need to be monitored and treated in the ICU for long periods of time.

> **Donna:** *Sharon has really made a lot of progress. At the beginning of her therapy, they asked her some questions or told her to put a dot in the middle of the paper. She could barely do any of this, she didn't have the control to do it. Her left arm was bent and paralyzed and she had to do everything with her right arm. She was barely able to hold a pencil and she could hardly write, but now she can write letters!*

It is difficult to predict the long-term symptoms after a severe head injury. At the worst extreme the patient may remain comatose or be totally dependent on others for self-care and mobility issues. Typically, the survivor of a severe head injury has a combination of long term-cognitive and physical problems that require continued assistance from others.

Overall, the prognosis for complete functional recovery is much less than for those who have sustained mild injuries. Functional recovery means the ability to return to a completely independent life. The long-term prognosis is also generally related to the length of time the patient was unconsciousness. The longer the amount of time spent in this state, the less functional recovery is observed.

For the family members of the severe head injury survivor it is important to remember that their loved one will require the long-term help of rehabilitation professionals to achieve as much independence as possible. The initial acute inpatient rehabilitation goals may be limited to preparing the patient and family members for long-term rehabilitation and teaching the family how to care for someone who has sustained a severe brain injury.

In between the mild and severe injuries are all the other injuries that are impossible to generalize or label. Patients with moderate injuries tend to require aggressive acute inpatient rehabilitation, just as intensively as those who sustain more severe injuries. They may also require ongoing long-term or outpatient therapy. The prognosis for functional recovery again depends on what areas of the brain have been affected. With more moderate injuries, the survivor may need to focus on specific areas like ambulation, self care, or memory instead of the more global problems of the severe brain injuries.

Is there any treatment for the personality/behavior problems associated with a frontal lobe injury?

Frontal lobe injuries can produce a wide variety of personality and behavior alterations. The degree and severity of these changes vary from patient to patient. Thankfully, multiple rehabilitation programs are available that can address these issues. Many of these programs combine occupational, physical, behavioral, and speech therapies to get these patients back to a functional status within society. The success of this therapy depends on the degree of abnormality present as a result of the injury. Family members should be braced for a fairly long road to recovery, keeping in mind that a complete return to the characteristics a patient had prior to the accident may not occur. Patience and understanding go a long way to aid in the recovery and rehabilitation process.

CHAPTER
13

⤜⤙•⤚⤛

Rites of Passage: A Spiritual Perspective on Rehabilitation

Rev. Scott K. Davis, M.Div.

T he time in the acute care hospital probably has been marked by profound and vivid physical, emotional, spiritual, and social experiences. With the announcement that the traumatic brain injury patient is ready to move to a rehabilitation setting, there may be a paradoxical feeling of joyous celebration and panicked anxiety. On the one hand, the transfer to a rehabilitation facility affirms what the patient and family members have been sensing about the improving physical, mental, and emotional states of the patient. The first part of the healing journey through days of uncertainty and despair seems to have passed, and hope appears to be glimmering on the horizon. But with the joy and relief comes some panic and fear. Moving to the rehabilitation setting, the uncertainty of expectations and outcomes returns. This anxiety is *déja vu*, similar to what patient and family members experienced in those first days in the acute care setting.

One way to consider what is happening dynamically and spiritually for patient and family in the movement to and through the rehabilitation setting is to see the process as a "rite of passage." Rites of passage are patterned ways in which persons and groups seek to describe and define personal crises of meaning as they affect the whole being of body-mind-spirit as well as relationships. Rites of passage are sacred journeys by which persons journey from the familiar and secure to the unfamiliar and unknown, resulting in personal change and new visions or directions for living. Three phases may be described in a rite of passage: separation, betwixt and between, and transformation.[1-3] Separation is a dramatic break from the old and familiar and the start of something new and different. In the betwixt and between phase, one endures a time of testing and discovery of who the person might become anew. With transformation, the person claims a new identity and role in the community. Celebrations commonly mark the beginning or end of the phases. A wedding ceremony, a graduation, a retirement party, a bar mitzvah, or confirmation are all celebrations of familiar rites of passage.

Separation is experienced as the patient and family members move from the predictable pattern of visitation, the personalities of the staff, and the daily routine of the acute hospital setting. Leaving the hospital marks a time of saying good-bye to nurses, doctors, social workers, therapists, and housekeepers. This may be a sad time, a time of grieving the loss of relationships through which healing was accomplished. It may be a joyous time of stories shared between staff, family members, and patient. Perhaps the family members or the staff will mark the occasion for the patient with a ritual—a party or informal send-off. Cards, pictures, flowers, and personal items are packed away for the trip to the rehabilitation setting. The point is that the acute care hospital is now passed, and the patient with the family members are being separated from it in order to move on. Generally, the patient is transported in special fashion to the new setting by means of wheelchair and ambulance.

At the new environment at the rehabilitation facility, the separation phase continues as the patient and family members submit to new rules and the expectations of the rehabilitation staff and facility. Visiting hours may differ, the therapy schedule may be more intense, the patient may be asked to do more independently. Being asked to trust new persons and new expectations in order to bring about further healing may evoke resistance, withdrawal, or hostility, as well as willing submission and acceptance. What is clear in this phase of separation is that the patient is in a strange place in order to become a person who is able to function as independently as possible in the community. One reminder of this goal is that patients are asked to dress as if they were in the community again and asked to eat in a common dining area. As alone as the patient may feel from loved ones, the patient is brought together in the rehabilitation facility with others who are struggling with similar physical, emotional, and spiritual issues in order to return to their family and community as a renewed, independent-as-possible person.

Scriptural stories about being separated from one's community may be encouraging during this phase. This can be a time of spiritual despair: feeling cut off, abandoned, lost, and hopeless. A key question for the patient to significant others may be, "Will you stay with me through this?" Biblical themes of exile and wilderness emphasize both the pain and struggle of being alone, as well as a trust and faith in someone/something needed beyond oneself in order to be sustained in the process.[4]

Separated from responsibilities at home and the care of loved ones, the individual can focus in this phase on the task of rehabilitative therapies. In the second phase in a rite of passage, betwixt and between, the individual is neither defined by one's old identity or abilities nor by any newly forged identity or capacities. The patient is not what he or she was (in terms of physical and/or mental capacities) and not yet what he or she might become through rehabilitative therapies. Traditionally, the betwixt and between phase is marked by tests of strength, endurance, courage, and faith. What a unique way of describing what the patient experiences in the course of therapies! It may be a time of doubting and questioning of one's present and future, or a reflective period of reorganizing one's priorities and values.[5] The patient may be asking God, "Why me?

Why now?" To significant others, the questions may be, "Will you accept me as I am (not as you wish me to be)?" "Will you help me in my quest toward independent living?" The patient may ask himself or herself: "Do you trust God, others, the process?" "Is this worth it?" This phase of transition often marks a time of a personal encounter with the spiritual. Through this encounter, an individual may recognize that one is not in control of life, but in relation to a larger (spiritual) force at work in the world.[6] The outcome is the discovery or rediscovery of the kind of person the individual wishes to be, buoyed by a spiritual story to guide the rehabilitation process into the final phase. Religious ritual and celebrations may underscore the spiritual work done by the individual in this phase. Confession and forgiveness, a commitment or recommitment to religious life, or increased interest in prayer, sacred text, and worship may emerge from this betwixt and between phase.

The final phase in the rite of passage as applied to rehabilitation is transformation. What was becoming apparent in the end of the previous phase continues to emerge with greater clarity and vision. As the length of stay in the rehabilitation facility concludes, the patient has gained a sense of *who* he or she is as a result of the traumatic brain injury as well as *what* he or she is capable of doing. In the course of the hospitalization and rehabilitation, the patient, along with the family members, has come face to face with the finite nature of bodily life and death, as well as the passing of one's identity as defined by physical, emotional, mental, spiritual, and social capacities. The rite of passage has produced a new person with a new vision for living. The individual has been transformed by the total experience and returns to the community different than when he or she left those many weeks or months before.[7] There is a new sense of vocation, a new perspective, and a new meaning about living and about relationships. Those who celebrate the transformation often express gratitude and the desire to share the experience with others.

And with the completion of the transformation phase, so begins the cycle of the rite of passage again. The good-byes at the rehabilitation facility mean that separation is at hand, and the trip home inaugurates the betwixt and between phase of adjusting to a once-familiar setting that may seem very new or different than one remembered it. And perhaps, the rite of passage back home will be marked with a ritual—a party, a gathering of friends, a welcome to the patient who moved from hospital to rehabilitation to home!

REFERENCES

1. Katonah J. Hospitalization: A rite of passage. In Holst LE, ed. Hospital Ministry: The Role of the Chaplain Today. New York: Crossroad, 1991, pp 55-67.
2. Anderson H, Foley E. Experiences in need of ritual. Christian Century, November 5, 1997, pp 1002-1008.
3. Carson TL. Liminal Reality and Transformational Power. New York: University Press of America, 1997.
4. Lamentations 3; Psalms 22 and 137; the temptation of Jesus in Matthew 4: 1-11.
5. The "dry bones" passage in Ezekiel 37; Psalm 131; Matthew 6:25-34.
6. Psalm 139; Job 38-42.
7. Jacob's transformation in Genesis 32:22-32.

CHAPTER
14

Afterword:
Head Injury Prevention

Despite all of the advanced technology available to physicians today, brain trauma is one of the leading causes of death and disability in the United States. The sheer number of people, particularly younger patients, affected by brain injury each year is staggering. Many patients are left severely debilitated, vegetative, or even dead from their brain injuries. Again, many of the patients are young, leaving both their lives and the lives of their loved ones permanently damaged. Although medical and surgical treatments for head injury have saved many lives over the years, even more patients cannot or do not benefit from the presently available therapies. In addition, while lives may be saved, the quality of the preserved life can at times be much less than satisfactory. The technology required to reverse all the damage done by traumatic brain injury simply does not exist at the present time. The brain does not heal and recover from injury as well as other parts of the body. When the brain is damaged, the injury often causes severe and irreversible problems. Therefore, as a society, we must try to implement the only treatment that is 100% effective. That treatment is prevention. Only by preventing the brain from being injured will we be able to rid society of the devastation caused by traumatic brain injury. There is no way to eliminate brain injury completely, but some very simple things can be done to help decrease the numbers of patients and families torn apart by this tragedy.

The use of alcohol and drugs is one of the most commonly seen factors in accidents leading to head injury. In many instances the head injury victim is not necessarily the individual who was using the mind-altering substance. In a motor vehicle accident, it is not uncommon for the intoxicated driver to be uninjured while the passenger suffers a devastating injury. In recent studies, alcohol was involved in 72% of the accidents that resulted in significant brain injury.[1] Clearly, by eliminating drunk driving and illegal drug use, we could dramatically decrease the number of head injuries. Imagine a physician who discovered a pill that could prevent 72% of all heart attacks. Withholding this medicine from the public would be considered a gross injustice. Now consider that people who have been convicted of drunk driving still operate motor vehicles in your community. The best treatment for head injury lies in the hands of all of us. Only through combined community effort with stronger laws, increased awareness, and a personal commitment toward responsible driving will we be able to significantly curb the incidence of head injuries in this country.

Obviously, preventing all head injuries is not a realistically attainable goal, but there are some simple ways to decrease their number and severity. Aside from drunk driving, other major contributing factors are domestic violence, work-related injuries, suicide, falls, and sports injuries. Federal and state governments can affect change by lowering speed limits, instituting mandatory seat belt laws, and impose harsh penalties for drunk drivers. Communities can affect change by supporting law enforcement agencies in their fight against drugs and violent crime. Families can take steps to ensure their own safety by using seat belts, buying cars with airbags, and wearing protective head gear when riding bikes. Keeping physically fit and wearing the proper equipment are ways to help decrease the severity and frequency of sports-related injuries. Companies have a responsibility to their employees to ensure a safe work environment. These companies should have regular safety checks and strictly enforced guidelines to help workers remain safe while on the job. There is no way to completely eliminate head injury but hopefully, through education and the simple rule of thinking before acting, we can reduce the significant impact that traumatic brain injury has on our society.

Ellen: Steve wasn't wearing a seat belt and that amazes me, because that was the biggest rule around our house. The car didn't move unless everyone was buckled up. Maybe he was so excited about his new job he just forgot. . . . They said there was a very slim chance that he had been wearing it and it came loose, but . . . He wasn't actually thrown from the car. He was hanging out the front passenger window laying on his back throwing up. He could have choked to death. The people who witnessed the accident said that he was like a rag doll bouncing back and forth in the car. He hit the median once, spun the car around, and hit it again, spun the car around, hit it again. Three times and he was just back and forth across the front seat.

———— ❧ COMMONLY ASKED QUESTIONS ❧ ————

If the patient had been wearing a seat belt, would the injury have been less severe?

Studies have suggested that wearing a seat belt does help to minimize injury severity sustained in motor vehicle accidents. While there is no way to tell for certain if a patient's injury would have been less severe if a seat belt had been worn, patients involved in motor vehicle accidents are more likely to strike the windshield, dashboard, or steering wheel when a seat belt is not worn. Extensive facial fractures, severe closed head injury, or significant internal organ damage can be the result of such impacts. Further, patients without a seat belt on can be thrown from the vehicle during an accident. In this situation, where the patient is no longer protected by the vehicle, the patient is exposed to significantly greater forces than those individuals who remain within the vehicle. The severity of injury is thus increased as is the likelihood of death. This is one reason why the law in many states requires that seat belts be worn at all times when traveling in a vehicle.

What can be done to prevent head injuries?

Many of the head injuries we see each year are the result of careless or dangerous behavior. Drunk driving, driving at high speeds, falls, and sports injuries are some of the more common sources of head injury. Many times people are injured because they do not take proper safety precautions or do things that impair their ability to make sound decisions.

As a community, we need to raise the general awareness of the devastating effects of brain injury on our society. Also, task forces against drunk driving are a simple but effective way of curtailing the incidence of driving-related head injury. One should keep in mind that alcohol plays a role in approximately 70% of all accidents resulting in brain injury. Employers and workers need to work together to ensure job safety through education and prevention programs. Schools, coaches, and athletes need to take proper precautions to ensure safety in the sports arena.

Is there anything we (the family members) could have done after the injury to prevent it from getting worse?

For a family confronted with an accident resulting in a major injury the best thing to do is to call for help as soon as possible. Above all else, time is the major factor that significantly impacts trauma victims. Family members or other bystanders at the scene of an accident should call 911 as soon as possible. The sooner a patient can receive treatment, the better the chances are for recovery. However, some injuries are so severe that it makes little difference when the treatments are initiated. Some patients sustain so much damage that there will be no chance for survival or recovery. In addition to obtaining prompt care, family members can also help to prevent secondary injury to the patient. Since head injury patients are at risk for cervical spine injuries, they should not be moved at all (unless the location is dangerous to the patient, such as near a fire) until the emergency crew arrives. Blankets can be used to keep the patient warm and pressure should be applied to any area of active bleeding. If the patient is not breathing, CPR should be initiated until help arrives.

Other things that are helpful for the physician are watching for seizures or any other abnormal movements. Providing emergency medical services (EMS) workers with a list of the patient's medications, allergies, and medical history is very important. Also report drug or alcohol use to the EMS worker because these substances can seriously compromise certain medical therapies. If the physician knows about them ahead of time, it helps in treating the patient more effectively and more safely.

REFERENCE

1. Kraus JF. Epidemiology of Head Injury. In Cooper PR, ed. Head Injury, 3rd ed. Baltimore: Williams & Wilkins, 1993, pp 1-25.

Glossary of Medical Terms

acute inpatient rehabilitation   A rehabilitation facility where the patient is admitted and receives an intense, multidisciplinary approach to therapy.

amnesia   The inability to remember events immediately before or after an injury.

anesthesiologist   A physician specialized in keeping a patient under paralysis and sedation through the use of special medications; many also specialize in the treatment of critically ill patients.

angiogram   A diagnostic test where dye is injected into the cerebral arteries and veins. X-ray films are then taken to visualize of the cerebral vascular anatomy; various interventions can also be performed during this procedure if necessary.

anterior cerebral artery   A branch of the internal carotid artery; it supplies blood to a portion of the frontal lobes, including the part that controls leg movements.

anticonvulsants   Medicines given to stop and control seizures; some common anticonvulsants are Dilantin (phenytoin), phenobarbital and Tegretol (carbamazepine).

antihypertensives   Medicines used to lower high blood pressure.

aphasias   Different types of speech abnormalities, including the inability to understand speech as well as the inability to speak correctly.

apraxia   Difficulty executing a particular motor task; more a planning problem in the brain than a weakness problem.

arterial blood gas (ABG)   Measurement of the oxygen content in a patient's arterial blood.

arterial line   A catheter inserted into an artery that enables continuous monitoring of blood pressure; these can also be used to draw blood from the patient, particularly for arterial blood gas determinations.

ascending reticular activating system (ARAS)   The system, which runs through the upper portions of the brain stem, involved in maintaining consciousness; acts to stimulate the brain and keep the patient awake. Injuries that involve this system can produce unconsciousness.

aspirate   The act of having oral secretions travel down the windpipe and into the lungs; see also *aspiration pneumonia*.

aspiration pneumonia   A lung infection frequently encountered in head injury patients; it results from oral secretions entering the windpipe and getting trapped in the lung. These secretions contain bacteria that can grow in the lung and cause a severe pneumonia.

ataxia   Instability and in-coordination when at rest or when attempting to move; typically secondary to damage to the cerebellum.

autonomic nervous system   A subdivision of our nervous system that is controlled by the brain stem. This system controls all the automatic functions of our body. These are the things our body does without us having to think about them. Examples include breathing, making our heart beat, and regulating temperature.

basilar artery   Formed by the joining of the two vertebral arteries, this artery is the main blood supply to the brain stem.

blood transfusion   Procedure in which matched blood is given to a patient intravenously. This is done for patients who have lost blood due to trauma or patients who are anemic.

bone flap   The "puzzle-piece" of bone removed from the skull by the neurosurgeon during a craniotomy.

brain death   A condition where the patient exhibits no evidence of any brain function. This is irreversible, and although the heart may still be beating, the patient is technically considered deceased.

brain parenchyma   The actual tissue that makes up the brain.

brain stem   The "stem" upon which the brain sits; it forms the connection between the brain and the spinal cord. It contains multiple fibers running to and from the brain, as well as the life control center for the body. It is divided into three portions: the midbrain, pons, and medulla.

Camino monitor   A fiberoptic cable placed through the skull to monitor the intracranial pressure. The tip of the cable lies just beneath the dura in the subdural space.

catheter   Another name for a tube; these are used to remove fluids from different areas of the body or to administer medications. Examples of catheters are the Foley catheter, an intravenous catheter, and a ventriculostomy.

cerebellum   The portion of the brain located underneath the occipital lobes. It is here that balance and coordination for the body are controlled.

cerebral aqueduct   A small canal that connects the third and fourth ventricles. If this canal becomes occluded, cerebrospinal fluid builds up in the rest of the ventricular system and results in hydrocephalus.

cerebral edema   The swelling (edema) that can occur in the brain (cerebral) secondary to various types of injury.

cerebrospinal fluid (CSF) The fluid that is made by the brain inside the ventricles. The fluid percolates through the inside of the brain and spinal cord and then flows out and over the top of both structures. The result is a protective, nutrient fluid layer that coats the brain and spinal cord on the inside and outside.

cerebrum Commonly referred to as the brain; it has two sides, a left and right side, with each side divided into portions called lobes.

cervical spine The region of the spinal cord directly below the brain. The cervical spinal cord is protected by the cervical spine, a series of ring-like bones. These bones are often broken in patients with head injury. Injury to the cervical spinal cord may cause paralysis.

chemical pneumonitis Patients with head injury often throw up. If the vomitus is aspirated, it can cause a severe chemical reaction in the lungs. This reaction resembles pneumonia but is not caused by bacteria and is not an infection. The patient generally improves with breathing treatments and ventilatory support.

choroid plexus The structures within the ventricles that actually make the cerebrospinal fluid.

closed head injury An injury to the brain in which the skull remains intact.

cognition The higher thought processes controlled within the brain. These include memory, speech, behavior, and personality. The Rancho Los Amigos scale is one method used to characterize cognitive deficits.

coma Description of a person's state of consciousness; a coma is said to exist when the person's level of consciousness is such that he or she is unable to purposefully interact with their environment.

comatose Any patient in a state of altered mental status such that he or she is unable to purposefully interact with their surroundings.

computed tomography (CT) scan A machine that uses x-rays to create detailed images of the brain; this machine is extremely useful in diagnosing and managing head injury.

conjugate gaze The eyes moving exactly in tandem as they move from side to side; damage to the centers that control this can result in double vision as the images collected by the two eyes are not perfectly aligned.

contracture Permanent fixation of a limb in a particular position; this can be the result of increased tone in patients with brain or spinal cord injury. Passive range-of-motion exercises attempt to prevent contractures from occurring.

convexity of the skull The area of the skull that would be covered by a baseball hat.

corneal reflex A protective reflex controlled by the pons in the brain stem; any irritation of the cornea (the clear surface of the eye) automatically results in blinking of the eye. The presence or absence of this reflex is used to determine the relative health of the pons.

corpus callosum The major connection between the two cerebral hemispheres. This structure enables the different lobes located on both sides of the brain to communicate with each other.

cranioplasty An operation in which the original bone flap, or a synthetic covering, is placed over the area where the initial craniotomy was performed. This is done for cosmetic purposes.

craniotomy General term for an operative procedure performed on the patient's head/brain.

crossed The manner in which most functions controlled by the brain are organized; the right side of the brain controls the left side of the body and vice versa.

DDAVP A drug given to a patient who has diabetes insipidus; this medicine signals the kidney to hold onto water molecules. After getting this drug the amount of urine the patient produces markedly decreases and becomes more concentrated.

decerebrate posture An abnormal reflex motor response caused by compression of the brain stem. The patient makes reflex movements in which the legs are vigorously straightened and the arms and hands are straight and turn inwardly. This is a reflexive response, in that the patient is comatose and not willfully performing the action.

decorticate posture An abnormal reflex motor response caused by compression of the midbrain. The patient reflexively straightens the legs and the arms curl up toward the head. This is an involuntary response, in that the patient is not willfully performing the action. Decorticate posturing is a better clinical sign than decerebrate posturing, but neither tends to be good.

deep vein thromboses (DVT) Blood clots that form in the large veins of the legs and pelvis. These clots may break off and float through the heart and into the lungs; see also *pulmonary embolism*.

diabetes insipidus (DI) A syndrome in head injury patients that causes them to lose a lot of water in the urine. The brain is unable to properly tell the kidney to hold on to water. This results in the patient producing a large amount of very diluted urine. Generally, this development in head injury patients is a sign of serious injury and correlates with a poor prognosis.

Dilantin (phenytoin) An anticonvulsant medication frequently used in head injury patients.

dilate An anatomic structure increasing in size; may refer to any hollow structure such as arteries, veins, ventricles, or bowels. The walls of the structure expand and thereby increase the size of the hollow area, similar to a balloon being blown up.

disseminated intravascular coagulation (DIC) A disorder of the body's clotting system; may develop in patients who have severe head injury or certain infections. This is a very serious life-threatening condition.

Dobhoff tube A thin tube placed in the nose or mouth and passed down the esophagus and into the stomach. It is used to give the patient medicines, water, and food.

dolls eyes response A test done to evaluate the patient's level of coma. The head is rotated from side to side as the movements of the eyes are recorded. The eyes should move in a certain way. If they fail to move an injury to the brain stem is likely.

dominant The side of the brain responsible for speech function. Close to 100% of right-handed patients and most left-handed patients have speech function controlled by the left side of the brain.

dura mater or **dura** A tough connective tissue membrane that surrounds the brain. Contained within the dura are the brain and cerebrospinal fluid.

dysarthria Difficulty speaking; words are typically slurred.

dysconjugate gaze The eyes, as they move from side to side, do not move exactly in tandem; can result in double vision in patients who are conscious.

dysphagia Difficulty swallowing, which can lead to unwanted aspiration and subsequent pneumonia.

edema Generalized term for swelling.

EEG A machine that measures brain activity by measuring the electrical brain waves. This machine can determine whether the patient is having seizures.

EKG A test that provides the physician with an electrical profile of the heart. It is useful in diagnosing heart attacks and arrhythmias.

EKG leads The small electrodes that are placed on the patient's chest and hooked up to the machine that produces the EKG.

electrolytes The molecules in our blood that provide the cells of the body with the things they need to function. Examples are sodium, potassium, and chloride.

emboli A piece of a blood clot that breaks off and flows into an artery or vein causing a block in that artery or vein.

emergency medical service (EMS) The paramedics who are usually first at the accident scene. They are skilled at stabilizing the patient and rapidly transporting the patient to the hospital.

endotracheal tube A tube placed in the trachea to protect the airway and to allow the ventilator to deliver breaths directly into the lungs.

epidural hematoma A collection of blood between the skull and dura (i.e., "outside" the brain).

esophagus The passageway that connects the mouth with the stomach.

evaporated Water changing from liquid to gas form. This can be appreciated by considering a pot of coffee. As the coffee sits on the stove, the water evaporates and the coffee gets progressively stronger in flavor as the concentration increases.

extending A type of posturing movement in which the patient rigidly straightens the arms and legs in response to a stimulus. This represents the worst type of posturing movement because it indicates that the damaged area in the brain stem is very close to the life control center.

extubation or **extubated** The act of removing the endotracheal tube from a patient. Once extubated, patients breathe on their own without assistance.

flexing A posturing response; the patient rigidly straightens out the legs and bends the arms at the elbows (i.e., flexes the arms). This is considered a better sign than an extending response.

Foley catheter A catheter inserted into the bladder; used to accurately measure the amount of urine produced and to prevent urine from getting on patients who are unconscious.

fourth ventricle The lowest portion of the ventricular system. It is a single ventricle located in the posterior fossa. It is the last stop for the cerebrospinal fluid before it drains out of the brain and enters the space around the spinal cord.

frontal lobes The paired lobes located in the front of the brain. Functions located in these lobes include movement, speech, emotion, motivation, and personality.

gag reflex This reflex occurs when the back of the throat is irritated. The resulting response helps to keep food and liquid out of the airway. This reflex is controlled by centers located in the medulla and its presence or absence can be used to determine the relative health of this structure.

Glasgow Coma Scale (GCS) A system used to grade the severity of a patient's head injury. The scale is based solely on the findings of the physician's neurologic examination of the patient. The scale ranges from 3 to 15 with 3 being the worst.

grand mal seizure A seizure that produces unconsciousness and uncontrollable shaking all over the body; can be very dangerous to the patient if they occur continuously and without interruption.

hematocrit A measurement of the concentration of red cells in the patient's blood. A drop in the hematocrit can sometimes indicate blood loss from bleeding.

hemianopsia Inability to see one full half of the visual field when looking straight ahead; can occur from damage to one occipital lobe.

hemiparesis   Weakness present on one side of the body; see also *hemiplegia*.

hemiplegia   Inability to move one side of the body, sometimes including the face; can occur from damage to the frontal lobe on the opposite side or the brain stem.

hemispheres   The two sides of the cerebral cortex. The cerebral cortex is made up of a right hemisphere and a left hemisphere.

hemodynamic profile   A set of numbers that measures a patient's heart and lung function; requires the use of indwelling monitors such as the Swan-Ganz catheter and arterial line.

herniation   A process in which the brain is pushed out of its normal position; can lead to compression of vital areas of the brain and cause rapid death.

hydrocephalus   A condition where the ventricular system begins to abnormally dilate, causing increased pressure within the brain.

hyperventilation   Using a ventilator to make the patient breathe rapidly. This makes the body breathe off more carbon dioxide that, in turn, lowers intracranial pressure.

hypotension   Very low blood pressure; usually of such a degree that blood flow to the brain is compromised.

hypoxia   A time period in which the brain does not receive oxygenated blood; can occur when the blood doesn't have enough oxygen (patient not breathing) or when the oxygenated blood doesn't reach the brain (severely low blood pressure).

inferior quadranopsia   Typically, secondary to parietal lobe injury, this deficit results in the inability to see the lower outer aspect of the visual field when looking straight ahead.

innervation   The control of a muscle by a specific nerve. Each muscle in our body moves according to the signals it gets from its supplying nerve. We say that the "nerve innervates the muscle."

intensive care unit (ICU)   A special location within the hospital where the sickest patients are admitted; where the most intense management for head injury occurs. Each room is equipped with special equipment to handle just about any medical situation.

internal carotid artery   Two arteries that deliver the main blood supply to the brain. Once within the brain, the carotid artery divides into smaller arteries that help supply blood to the brain.

internal carotid artery dissection   Usually results from trauma to the head or neck. A tear in the internal layer of the blood vessel that allows blood to track between the walls of the blood vessel; may lead to stroke.

intracerebral contusion   A bruising of a specific region of the brain from trauma to the head.

intracranial pressure (ICP)   The pressure within the head. The brain, blood, and the cerebrospinal fluid in the ventricles all contribute to the overall pressure.

intravenous lines (IV)   Small flexible catheters inserted into veins; can be used to administer fluids and medications directly into the bloodstream.

intubated   A person is considered "intubated" when a breathing tube (endotracheal tube) is placed within the patient's airway.

ischemia   A process in which an organ in the body does not receive the oxygen-rich blood it needs; caused by blockage of an artery that stops the oxygenated blood from reaching the brain. An example is a stroke.

isolated head injury   The head is injured but no other part of the body is hurt.

larynx   The part of the windpipe that contains the voice box; the structure in the neck commonly referred to as the Adam's apple.

lateral ventricle   The largest compartment of the ventricular system; there are two paired lateral ventricles within the brain that drain into the third ventricle.

localizing   Patients who move a limb, usually the hand, to the location where the stimulus is being applied; considered to be a better sign than patients who exhibit posturing responses.

long-term rehabilitation   A program typically used for patients with severe head injuries who require extensive and prolonged therapy over months or years.

lumen   The hollow part of a tube; for example, water running through a garden hose travels through a lumen.

magnetic resonance imaging (MRI)   A machine that produces extremely detailed pictures of all the different parts of the brain; it uses magnets instead of x-rays to create the pictures.

Mannitol   A drug used to lower intracranial pressure. This drug tends to decrease swelling by causing the body to lose water in the urine.

medulla   The lowest portion of the brain stem. The medulla contains the life control center, which controls the heart rate, breathing and blood pressure. The gag reflex is also controlled by the medulla.

meningitis   A serious infection involving the coverings of the brain. A spinal tap is generally needed to diagnose this potentially fatal disease.

midbrain   The uppermost part of the brain stem. The centers that control the size of the pupils are located here.

middle cerebral artery   A branch of the internal carotid artery; supplies blood to a large portion of the brain, including the areas that control movement, sensation, and speech.

motor activity   Describes the extent to which the patient is moving; included are the movements made in response to a stimulus as well as any spontaneous movements.

motor area   The regions in the cerebral cortex that control muscle movements of the body.

nasogastric (NG) tube   A tube placed in the nose and passed down the esophagus and into the stomach; can be used to suck material such as blood and air out of the stomach. These tubes can also be used to give medicines and feedings.

neglect   A patient ignores a part of the body; can appear to be an inability to move one side of the body and can occur with parietal lobe damage.

nervous system   A general term used to describe the brain, spinal cord, and nerves of the body.

neuron   A nerve cell; the most basic element of each member of the nervous system.

neurosurgeon   A physician who specializes in operative problems dealing with the nervous system; operates on the brain, spine, and nerves.

non-dominant   The side of the brain not responsible for speech function. In most patients, this is the right side of the brain.

Norcuron   A drug used by physicians to achieve total body paralysis; most commonly used by anesthesiologists on patients undergoing surgery. It has been effective in controlling elevated intracranial pressure in some head injury patients but must be used in combination with a sedating drug such as morphine.

nystagmus   Specific eye movements that appear with damage to specific sites of the brain. These eye movements may help the physician diagnose where the brain damage is located.

occipital lobes   Paired lobes, located in the back of the brain, that deal predominately with vision.

open head injury   An injury to the brain in which the skull is fractured and the overlying scalp is lacerated.

orthopedist (orthopedic surgeon)   A physician who specializes in bone and joint injuries.

outpatient rehabilitation   When the patient is discharged home and receives therapy at regularly scheduled appointments during the week; typically reserved for patients with minimal rehabilitation needs.

paralysis   An inability to move a portion of the body. This condition can involve a single limb, an entire side, or the whole body.

paralytics Medicines, such as Norcuron, used to induce total muscle paralysis in the body.

parietal lobes Located behind the frontal lobes and above the temporal lobes. The left parietal lobe typically deals with multiple language functions, including understanding speech, reading, and writing.

pentobarbital coma A drug places the patient in a state of suspended animation; dramatically lowers intracranial pressure but is associated with a high complication rate.

percutaneous endoscopic gastrostomy (PEG) A feeding tube surgically inserted through the abdominal wall into the stomach; more permanent than a Dobhoff or nasogastric tube. PEG tubes can be removed when no longer needed.

pericranium A thin layer of connective tissue that covers the outside of the skull; can be carefully removed from the skull and used to patch dural tears.

persistent vegetative state Results from severe brain injury. State in which there is a return of wakefulness but no sign of higher cortical function. The patients may appear to be awake but never regain conscious awareness.

phenytoin See *Dilantin*.

pneumatic air stockings Leg garments that sequentially inflate and deflate; these pumps help prevent deep vein thromboses.

pneumonia An infection in the lung; frequently occurs in head injury patients because of aspiration.

pneumothorax or **pneumothoraces** Collapsed lung; can be caused by rib fractures, after placement of central lines, or in any patient attached to a ventilator.

pons Located in the center of the brain stem; the location of various centers that help to control different functions, including facial sensation and movements.

posterior fossa Special compartment in the back of the skull just above where the skull and neck connect where the cerebellum is located.

posttraumatic seizures Convulsions that may develop after a brain injury; affect approximately 15% of all patients with brain injuries. Most achieve seizure control with anticonvulsant medication.

posturing Automatic or reflexive movements; occurs when the brain is no longer in control of the body and the brain stem takes over. This unveils the automatic movements controlled by the brain stem. Posturing movements include flexing and extending.

pulmonary artery One of the large arteries that brings blood from the heart to the lungs.

pulmonary embolism Blockage of a branch of the pulmonary artery from a blood clot; can cause severe breathing problems and even death.

pulse oximeter   A small monitoring device placed on the finger to monitor oxygen saturation of the blood.

pupillary reflex   The normal reaction of the black center of the eye to light; the pupil should shrink when light is shined into the eye.

purposeful   Patients who are not as deeply unconscious may exhibit movements that appear to be directed at accomplishing a particular goal. This sign suggests there is some brain activity involved in the movement.

seizure   Occurs when there is excessive and disorganized electrical activity in the brain. Patients may or may not exhibit movements or shaking during these events; damaged areas in the brain can irritate and "short circuit" the normal electrical activity within the brain.

sepsis   An infection in the body's bloodstream; very dangerous because the infection can spread anywhere in the body.

serum osmolarity   A blood test that monitors the concentration of the blood.

sputum   Oral secretions that build up in the lungs or endotracheal tube; must be frequently suctioned to keep the airway clean help prevent pneumonia from developing.

step-down unit   A section of the hospital that provides special intermediate care for patients; provides extra services for patients not quite ready for a regular hospital room.

subacute inpatient rehabilitation   A program where the patient is admitted and receives therapy; provides less intense therapy for patients who cannot tolerate the more intensive therapies provided in acute rehabilitation.

subarachnoid hemorrhage   Refers to blood within the spaces that the brain's blood vessels travel. This is typically diffuse.

subcutaneous heparin   A drug injected under the skin that helps prevent deep vein thromboses.

subdural hematoma   A collection of blood on the surface of the brain.

superior quadranopsia   The inability to see the upper outer aspect of the visual field when looking straight ahead; damage to either temporal lobe can produce such a visual deficit by affecting the connections that run from the eyes to the occipital lobes.

Swan-Ganz catheter   A special catheter passed down the large veins, through the heart, and into the larger vessels in the lungs. This multipurpose catheter helps to monitor various functions, including heart function, fluid status, and the pressure within the lungs.

syndrome of inappropriate antidiuretic hormone (SIADH)   A condition in which the kidney is unable to excrete water in the urine, essentially the exact opposite of diabetes insipidus.

systemic blood pressure   The force at which the heart pumps the blood through the body.

telemetry   Continuous monitoring of the electrical activity of the heart.

temporal lobes   The paired lobes located on the lower sides of the brain and closest to the brain stem. Functions in these lobes include memory and speech.

tentorium   The roof of the posterior fossa that separates the cerebellum from the rest of the brain; made of dura.

thalamus   The relay station between the brain and the rest of the body. Just about all the signals sent to the brain go through the thalamus before continuing on to the brain.

third nerve (oculomotor nerve)   A paired nerve that starts on either side of the midbrain and runs forward to each eye; controls the pupillary light response reflex.

third ventricle   A single, narrow ventricle found within the center of the brain. The lateral ventricles drain cerebrospinal fluid into it and, in turn, it drains into the fourth ventricle via the cerebral aqueduct.

trachea   The main passageway for air between the mouth and lungs; branches into smaller portions in the two lungs.

tracheostomy   A surgical procedure in which a small, rigid, plastic tube is placed directly into the trachea through the neck; helps to protect the airway while avoiding an endotracheal tube down the throat.

transcranial Doppler   A device that bounces sound waves off the blood vessels in the neck and brain; enables the determination of the individual blood flow characteristics within various vessels.

trauma surgeon   A physician specialized in treating patients with multiple traumatic injuries.

unconsciousness   A state in which the patient appears asleep. Although higher cortical function may not be present, patients may still respond to different stimuli. This can occur from simultaneous damage to both sides of the brain or injury to the brain stem.

urinary tract infections   An infection frequently seen in chronically sick patients in the intensive care unit setting. The risk of infection increases with continual use of a Foley catheter.

vasospasm   A reflexive response of blood vessels to damage. The arteries of the brain may constrict in response to head injury. This can lead to secondary hypoxic damage because when the blood vessels constrict they carry less blood to the brain.

ventilator   A machine that assists patients in breathing. Various settings on the ventilator can be adjusted, including the amount of oxygen in each breath, the depth or amount of each breath, and the number of breaths delivered each minute; is also known as a "respirator."

ventricular system or **ventricles**   The fluid-filled spaces within the brain that make and contain the cerebrospinal fluid. The fluid runs through this system and is ultimately absorbed back into the bloodstream. The ventricular system is composed of two lateral ventricles, a single third ventricle, and a single fourth ventricle.

ventriculoperitoneal (VP) shunt   A surgically implanted device that drains the cerebrospinal fluid within the ventricles internally into the abdomen via a soft tube.

ventriculostomy   A tube used to measure intracranial pressure and drain cerebrospinal fluid out of the brain. The tube is placed through a small hole in the skull and passed through the brain into the lateral ventricle.

vertebral arteries   These help to make up the secondary blood supply to the brain and brain stem. These join and form the basilar artery, which is the main blood supply to the brain stem.

vertebrobasilar system   Refers to the blood vessels that bring blood from the heart to the spinal cord, cerebellum, and brain stem; consists of the basilar and vertebral arteries.

visual system   The system that allows us to see. It is composed of the eyes, the occipital lobes, and the connections that run between these two structures. As with most functions controlled by the brain, this system is crossed so that one side of the brain controls vision for the opposite side.

vomitus   The material expelled when a person throws up.

weaning the patient from the ventilator   A process by which the breathing support given to the patient by the ventilator is gradually turned down; allows the patient to do more of the breathing and helps build up the lungs prior to extubation (removal of the breathing tube).

Index of Questions

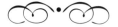

Chapter 4. Lab Work and Imaging

Chapter 5. Typical Symptoms and Behavior

Chapter 6. Surgical Management

Chapter 7. The Intensive Care Setting

Chapter 8. Other Medical Issues

Chapter 9. Prognosis and Outcomes

Additional Resources

Professional Societies

American Association of Neurological
Surgeons
22 South Washington Street
Park Ridge, IL 60068-4287
Phone: 847-692-9500
Fax: 847-692-6770

Congress of Neurological Surgeons
22 South Washington Street
Park Ridge, IL 60068-4287
Phone: 847-692-9500
Fax: 847-692-6770

American Academy of Neurology
1080 Montreal Avenue
St. Paul, MN 55116
Phone: 612-695-1940
Web site: http://www.aan.com

Society for Neuroscience
11 Dupont Circle, NW, Suite 500
Washington DC 20036
Phone: 202-462-6688
Web site: http://www.sfn.org

Support Organizations

Brain Injury Association, Inc. (BIA)
1776 Massachusetts Avenue NW, Suite 100
Washington, DC 20036-1904
Phone: 202-296-6443
Fax: 202-296-8850
Family Helpline: 800-444-6443
Web site: http://www.biausa.org
*The Brain Injury Association helps promote
awareness, understanding, and prevention of
brain injury through education, advocacy, and
community support services. Their web site has
links to state chapters, support groups, and a*
*wealth of information on various aspects of brain
injury. Call the Family Helpline for information
and referrals.*

International Brain Injury Association
(IBIA)
1776 Massachusetts Avenue NW, Suite 105
Washington, DC 20036-1904
Phone: 202-835-0580
Fax: 202-835-0584 or 703-758-0221
*The International Brain Injury Association's
mission is to provide worldwide leadership in pro-
moting programs, opportunities, and services for
those with brain injury.*

THINK FIRST Foundation
22 South Washington Street
Park Ridge, IL 60068
Phone: 847-692-2740
Web site: http://www.thinkfirst.org/home.
htm
*THINK FIRST has created a public education
program for teens and young adults for the prevention of head and spinal cord injury.*

Web Links

National Resource Center for Traumatic
Brain Injury
http://www.neuro.pmr.vcu.edu/LINKS/sup-
port.htm

The Brain Injury Ring
http://www.alliance.net/~jame/bir/bir.htm

The Perspectives Network
http://www.tbi.org

The ABI/TBI Information Project
http://www.sasquatch.com/tbi

Index

Notes

Notes

Notes

Notes